Medical Interpreter's Dictionary

Eric Engle

Copyright © 2024 Eric Engle

All rights reserved.

DEDICATION

For Hippocrates and Asclepius

Table of Contents
1. PATIENCE PATIENTS. THE HOSPITAL ROOM......................6
2. GIMME A BREAK. FRACTURES SPRAINS DISLOCATIONS.15
3. EYE ONLY HAVE EYES FOR YOU: EYE INJURIES 26
4. SHOW ME ON THE DOLLY: SYMPTOMATIC DESCRIPTIONS...30
5. SICK BURN! BURNS SCALDING AND BLISTERING...........42
6. CAN YOU STOMACH THIS? ESOPHAGAL INJURIES 51
7. COUGH IT UP! Terms related to symptoms of coughing: 61
8. HOSPITAL ROOM FURNITURE IN THE HOSPITAL.............73
9. BODY PLACES...123
10. SO HOT! FEVERS 157

ACKNOWLEDGMENTS

I just want to thank any medical personnel who have helped me when I was unwell. The best way to use this dictionary is to also get the eBook then you can search for terms more effectively and also have the manual easily at hand for you or your patient. I priced both as low as amazon allows so you can serve others well. Finally, if you medicos know friends into literature and languages key them in on medical interpreting, one can make a good living at that. Thanks!

1. PATIENCE PATIENTS. THE HOSPITAL ROOM

1. Bed (English) - Lit (French) - Cama (Spanish) - Bett (German) - Кровать (Russian) - 床 (Chuáng) (Mandarin)

   - Definition: A piece of furniture used for sleeping or resting.

2. Pillow (English) - Oreiller (French) - Almohada (Spanish) - Kissen (German) - Подушка (Russian) - 枕头 (Zhěntou) (Mandarin)

   - Definition: A cushioned support for the head during sleep or rest.

3. Blanket (English) - Couverture (French) - Manta (Spanish) - Decke (German) - Одеяло (Russian) - 毯子 (Tǎnzi) (Mandarin)

   - Definition: A large piece of fabric used to keep warm, usually on a bed.

4. Call button (English) - Bouton d'appel (French) - Botón de llamada (Spanish) - Rufknopf (German) - Кнопка вызова (Russian) - 呼叫按钮 (Hūjiào ànniǔ) (Mandarin)

   - Definition: A button that patients can press to call for assistance from hospital staff.

5. I.V. (intra-venous) pole (English) - Perche à perfusion (French) - Soporte de suero (Spanish) - Infusionsständer (German) - Стойка для капельницы (Russian) - 输液架 (Shūyè jià) (Mandarin)

   - Definition: A stand used to hang intravenous (IV) bags containing fluids or medications.

6. Wheelchair (English) - Fauteuil roulant (French) - Silla de ruedas (Spanish) - Rollstuhl (German) - Кресло-коляска (Russian) - 轮椅 (Lúnyǐ) (Mandarin)

   - Definition: A chair with wheels used for transporting patients who are unable to walk.

7. Blood pressure cuff (English) - Brassard de pression sanguine

(French) - Brazalete de presión arterial (Spanish) - Blutdruckmanschette (German) - Манжета для измерения давления (Russian) - 血压袖带 (Xuèyā xiùdài) (Mandarin)

   - Definition: A device wrapped around the arm to measure blood pressure.

8. Stethoscope (English) - Stéthoscope (French) - Estetoscopio (Spanish) - Stethoskop (German) - Стереофонендоскоп (Russian) - 听诊器 (Tīngzhěn qì) (Mandarin)

   - Definition: A medical instrument used to listen to sounds within the body, especially the heart and lungs.

9. Patient gown (English) - Chemise de patient (French) - Bata de paciente (Spanish) - Patientenhemd (German) - Халат пациента (Russian) - 病人服 (Bìngrén fú) (Mandarin)

   - Definition: Loose-fitting clothing worn by patients in hospitals or medical facilities.

10. Thermometer (English) - Thermomètre (French) - Termómetro (Spanish) - Thermometer (German) - Термометр (Russian) - 温度计 (Wēndù jì) (Mandarin)

    - Definition: A device used to measure body temperature.

11. Tray (English) - Plateau (French) - Bandeja (Spanish) - Tablett (German) - Лоток (Russian) - 托盘 (Tuōpán) (Mandarin)

    - Definition: A flat, shallow container used for holding items such as food, medications, or medical supplies.

12. Gown (English) - Robe (French) - Bata (Spanish) - Kittel (German) - Халат (Russian) - 长袍 (Chángpáo) (Mandarin)

    - Definition: A loose-fitting garment worn by healthcare professionals for hygiene and protection.

13. Scale (English) - Balance (French) - Báscula (Spanish) - Waage (German) - Весы (Russian) - 称 (Chèng) (Mandarin)

- Definition: A device used to measure weight.

14. Sphygmomanometer (English) - Sphygmomanomètre (French) - Esfigmomanómetro (Spanish) - Blutdruckmessgerät (German) - Сфигмоманометр (Russian) - 血压计 (Xiěyā jì) (Mandarin)

- Definition: A device used to measure blood pressure.

15. Examination table (English) - Table d'examen (French) - Mesa de examen (Spanish) - Untersuchungstisch (German) - Испытательный стол (Russian) - 检查台 (Jiǎnchá tái) (Mandarin)

- Definition: A table used by healthcare professionals to examine patients.

16. Hand sanitizer (English) - Gel hydroalcoolique (French) - Desinfectante de manos (Spanish) - Händedesinfektionsmittel (German) - Средство для обработки рук (Russian) - 洗手液 (Xǐshǒu yè) (Mandarin)

- Definition: A liquid or gel used to disinfect hands, often containing alcohol.

17. Urinal (English) - Urinal (French) - Orinal (Spanish) - Urinflasche (German) - Уринол (Russian) - 尿壶 (Niào hú) (Mandarin)

- Definition: A container used for urination when a patient is unable to use a toilet.

18. Waste bin (English) - Poubelle (French) - Papelera (Spanish) - Abfalleimer (German) - Мусорное ведро (Russian) - 垃圾桶 (Lèsè tǒng) (Mandarin)

- Definition: A container for disposing of waste materials.

19. Privacy curtain (English) - Rideau d'intimité (French) - Cortina de privacidad (Spanish) - Sichtschutzvorhang (German) - Занавеска для конфиденциальности (Russian) - 隔离帘 (Gélí lián) (Mandarin)

- Definition: A curtain used to provide privacy for patients during medical examinations or procedures.

20. Blood pressure measurement (English) - Mesure de la pression artérielle (French) - Medición de la presión arterial (Spanish) - Blutdruckmessung (German) - Измерение артериального давления (Russian) -

21. Oxygen mask (English) - Masque à oxygène (French) - Máscara de oxígeno (Spanish) - Sauerstoffmaske (German) - Маска для кислорода (Russian) - 氧气面罩 (Yǎngqì miànzhào) (Mandarin)

   - Definition: A mask that covers the nose and mouth to deliver oxygen to a patient's lungs.

22. Electrocardiogram (ECG or EKG) machine (English) - Appareil d'électrocardiogramme (French) - Electrocardiograma (Spanish) - EKG-Gerät (German) - Электрокардиограф (Russian) - 心电图机 (Xīndiàntú jī) (Mandarin)

   - Definition: A machine used to record the electrical activity of the heart.

23. Catheter (English) - Cathéter (French) - Catéter (Spanish) - Katheter (German) - Катетер (Russian) - 导管 (Dǎoguǎn) (Mandarin)

   - Definition: A thin tube inserted into the body to drain fluids or administer medication.

24. Nasogastric tube (NG tube) (English) - Sonde nasogastrique (French) - Sonda nasogástrica (Spanish) - Nasogastraler Schlauch (German) - Назогастральный зонд (Russian) - 鼻胃管 (Bí wèi guǎn) (Mandarin)

   - Definition: A tube inserted through the nose and into the stomach for feeding or drainage purposes.

25. Blood draw (English) - Prélèvement sanguin (French) - Extracción de sangre (Spanish) - Blutentnahme (German) - Взятие крови (Russian) - 抽血 (Chōu xiě) (Mandarin)

   - Definition: The process of taking a blood sample from a patient for testing or analysis.

26. Foley catheter (English) - Cathéter de Foley (French) - Sonda Foley (Spanish) - Foley-Katheter (German) - Катетер Фолея (Russian) - 弗利导尿管 (Fú lì dǎoniaò guǎn) (Mandarin)

   - Definition: A specialized urinary catheter that remains in the bladder to drain urine continuously.

27. Pulse oximeter (English) - Oxymètre de pouls (French) - Oxímetro de pulso (Spanish) - Pulsoximeter (German) - Пульсоксиметр (Russian) - 脉搏血氧饱和度仪 (Màibó xuèyǎng bǎohé dù yí) (Mandarin)

   - Definition: A device used to measure the oxygen saturation level in the blood.

28. Defibrillator (English) - Défibrillateur (French) - Desfibrilador (Spanish) - Defibrillator (German) - Дефибриллятор (Russian) - 除颤器 (Chúchàn qì) (Mandarin)

   - Definition: A device used to deliver an electric shock to the heart to restore normal rhythm in cases of cardiac arrest or arrhythmia.

29. Suction machine (English) - Aspirateur à succion (French) - Máquina de succión (Spanish) - Absauggerät (German) - Аспиратор (Russian) - 吸引机 (Xīyǐn jī) (Mandarin)

   - Definition: A device used to remove secretions, blood, or other fluids from a patient's airway or surgical site.

30. ECG leads (English) - Dérivations d'électrocardiogramme (French) - Electrodos de electrocardiograma (Spanish) - EKG-Elektroden (German) - Электроды ЭКГ (Russian) - 心电图导联 (Xīndiàntú dǎolián) (Mandarin)

   - Definition: Electrodes attached to the patient's skin to record the electrical activity of the heart.

31. Intravenous (IV) drip (English) - Perfusion intraveineuse

(French) - Goteo intravenoso (Spanish) - Intravenöser Tropf (German) - Внутривенное вливание (Russian) - 静脉滴注 (Jìngmài dīzhù) (Mandarin)

   - Definition: A method of delivering fluids, medications, or nutrients directly into a vein through a tube connected to an IV bag or pump.

32. Crash cart (English) - Chariot d'urgence (French) - Carro de paro (Spanish) - Notfallwagen (German) - Карета скорой помощи (Russian) - 急救车 (Jíjiù chē) (Mandarin)

   - Definition: A mobile cart stocked with emergency medical equipment and supplies used during resuscitation efforts or medical emergencies.

33. Specimen collection container (English) - Contenant de prélèvement (French) - Recipiente de recolección de muestras (Spanish) - Probenentnahmebehälter (German) - Емкость для сбора материала (Russian) - 标本收集容器 (Biāoběn shōují róngqì) (Mandarin)

   - Definition: A container used to collect and store biological samples such as urine, blood, or stool for laboratory analysis.

34. Crash trolley (English) - Chariot d'urgence (French) - Carro de paro (Spanish) - Notfallwagen (German) - Карета скорой помощи (Russian) - 急救推车 (Jíjiù tuīchē) (Mandarin)

   - Definition: A mobile cart equipped with emergency medical supplies and equipment used during critical situations or cardiac arrest.

35. Sterile gloves (English) - Gants stériles (French) - Guantes estériles (Spanish) - Sterile Handschuhe (German) - Стерильные перчатки (Russian) - 无菌手套 (Wújūn shǒutào) (Mandarin)

   - Definition: Gloves that have been sterilized to prevent contamination during medical procedures or patient care.

36. Privacy door (English) - Porte d'intimité (French) - Puerta de privacidad (Spanish) - Privatsphäre Tür (German) - Дверь для

конфиденциальности (Russian) - 隐私门 (Yǐnsī mén) (Mandarin)

   - Definition: A door used to ensure privacy for patients in hospital rooms or examination areas.

37. Examination light (English) - Lampe d'examen (French) - Luz de examen (Spanish) - Untersuchungsleuchte (German) - Осветительный прибор (Russian) - 检查灯 (Jiǎnchá dēng) (Mandarin)

   - Definition: A specialized light used by healthcare professionals to illuminate the area being examined during medical procedures or examinations.

38. Respiratory mask (English) - Masque respiratoire (French) - Mascarilla respiratoria (Spanish) - Atemschutzmaske (German) - Дыхательная маска (Russian) - 呼吸面罩 (Hūxī miànzhào) (Mandarin)

   - Definition: A mask worn over the nose and mouth to protect against inhalation of airborne particles or pathogens.

39. Sphygmomanometer cuff (English) - Brassard de sphygmomanomètre (French) - Brazalete de esfigmomanómetro (Spanish) - Blutdruckmanschette (German) - Манжета сфигмоманометра (Russian) - 血压计袖带 (Xiěyā jì xiùdài) (Mandarin)

   - Definition: The inflatable cuff used in conjunction with a sphygmomanometer to measure blood pressure.

40. Digital thermometer (English) - Thermomètre numérique (French) - Termómetro digital (Spanish) - Digitales Thermometer (German) - Цифровой термометр (Russian) - 数字温度计 (Shùzì wēndù jì) (Mandarin)

   - Definition: A thermometer that provides temperature readings electronically, typically through a digital display.

41. Portable oxygen concentrator (English) - Concentrateur

d'oxygène portable (French) - Concentrador de oxígeno portátil (Spanish) - Tragbarer Sauerstoffkonzentrator (German) - Портативный концентратор кислорода (Russian) - 便携式氧气浓缩器 (Biànxié shì yǎngqì nóngsuō qì) (Mandarin)

- Definition: A device that concentrates oxygen from the surrounding air for delivery to patients requiring supplemental oxygen therapy.

42. Foley catheter insertion (English) - Insertion de cathéter de Foley (French) - Inserción de sonda Foley (Spanish) - Einführung eines Foley-Katheters (German) - Введение катетера Фолея (Russian) - 弗利导尿管插入 (Fú lì dǎoniaò guǎn chārù) (Mandarin)

- Definition: The process of inserting a Foley catheter into the bladder through the urethra to drain urine.

43. Bedside commode (English) - Chaise percée (French) - Silla de ruedas con orinal (Spanish) - Toilettenstuhl (German) - Подмывное кресло (Russian) - 床边便椅 (Chuáng biān biànyǐ) (Mandarin)

- Definition: A portable chair with a toilet seat and a removable container used for toileting when a patient is unable to use a regular toilet.

44. Nebulizer (English) - Nébuliseur (French) - Nebulizador (Spanish) - Vernebler (German) - Небулайзер (Russian) - 雾化器 (Wùhuà qì) (Mandarin)

- Definition: A device that converts liquid medication into a fine mist for inhalation, commonly used to deliver respiratory medications.

45. Leg compression device (English) - Dispositif de compression des jambes (French) - Dispositivo de compresión de piernas (Spanish) - Beinkompressionsgerät (German) - Устройство для компрессии ног (Russian) - 腿部压力装置 (Tuǐbù yālì zhuāngzhì) (Mandarin)

- Definition: A device that applies intermittent pressure to the legs to prevent blood clots and promote circulation, often used during surgery or periods of immobility.

46. Personal protective equipment (PPE) (English) - Équipement de protection individuelle (EPI) (French) - Equipo de protección personal (EPP) (Spanish) - Persönliche Schutzausrüstung (PSA) (German) - Средства индивидуальной защиты (СИЗ) (Russian) - 个人防护装备 (Gèrén fánghù zhuāngbèi) (Mandarin)

   - Definition: Protective clothing, masks, gloves, and other equipment worn to minimize exposure to infectious agents or hazardous substances.

47. IV catheter insertion (English) - Insertion de cathéter intraveineux (French) - Inserción de catéter intravenoso (Spanish) - Einführung eines intravenösen Katheters (German) - Введение интравенозного катетера (Russian) - 静脉导管插入 (Jìngmài dǎoguǎn chārù) (Mandarin)

   - Definition: The process of inserting an intravenous catheter into a vein for the administration of fluids, medications, or blood products.

48. Pulse oximetry monitoring (English) - Monitorage de la saturation en oxygène (French) - Monitorización de la saturación de oxígeno (Spanish) - Pulsoxymetrie-Überwachung (German) - Мониторинг насыщения кислородом (Russian) - 脉搏血氧监测 (Màibó xuèyǎng jiāncè) (Mandarin)

   - Definition: Continuous monitoring of oxygen saturation levels in the blood using a pulse oximeter.

49. Wound dressing change (English) - Changement de pansement de plaie (French) - Cambio de apósito de herida (Spanish) - Wundverbandwechsel (German) - Смена повязки на ране (Russian) - 伤口敷料更换 (Shāngkǒu fūliào gēnghuàn) (Mandarin)

   - Definition: The process of removing and replacing the dressing on a wound to promote healing and prevent infection.

50. Rehabilitation exercises (English) - Exercices de rééducation (French) - Ejercicios de rehabilitación (Spanish) - Rehabilitationsübungen (German) - Упражнения по реабилитации

(Russian) - 康复锻炼 (Kāngfù duànliàn) (Mandarin)

   - Definition: Physical exercises or therapy sessions aimed at restoring function, strength, and mobility after injury or illness.

2. GIMME A BREAK. FRACTURES SPRAINS DISLOCATIONS.

1. Fracture (English) - Fracture (French) - Fractura (Spanish) - Fraktur (German) - Перелом (Russian) - 骨折 (Gǔzhé) (Mandarin)

   - Definition: A break or crack in a bone.

2. Sprain (English) - Entorse (French) - Esguince (Spanish) - Verstauchung (German) - Растяжение (Russian) - 扭伤 (Niǔshāng) (Mandarin)

   - Definition: An injury to a ligament caused by stretching or tearing.

3. Dislocation (English) - Luxation (French) - Luxación (Spanish) - Luxation (German) - Вывих (Russian) - 脱位 (Tuōwèi) (Mandarin)

   - Definition: The displacement of a bone from its normal position within a joint.

4. Avulsion fracture (English) - Fracture par arrachement (French) - Fractura por avulsión (Spanish) - Abrissfraktur (German) - Отрывной перелом (Russian) - 撕脱性骨折 (Sītuō xìng gǔzhé) (Mandarin)

   - Definition: A fracture where a small piece of bone is pulled away from the main bone due to the force of a tendon or ligament.

5. Greenstick fracture (English) - Fracture en bois vert (French) - Fractura en tallo verde (Spanish) - Grünholzfraktur (German) - Перелом зеленой ветви (Russian) - 绿枝骨折 (Lǜ zhī gǔzhé) (Mandarin)

   - Definition: A fracture where the bone is partially broken, resembling a green branch that has been bent but not completely snapped.

6. Spiral fracture (English) - Fracture en spirale (French) - Fractura espiral (Spanish) - Spiralfraktur (German) - Спиральный перелом (Russian) - 螺旋骨折 (Luóxuán gǔzhé) (Mandarin)

   - Definition: A fracture that occurs in a twisting pattern along the length of the bone.

7. Boxer's fracture (English) - Fracture du boxeur (French) - Fractura del boxeador (Spanish) - Boxerfraktur (German) - Перелом боксера (Russian) - 拳击手骨折 (Quánjí shǒu gǔzhé) (Mandarin)

   - Definition: A fracture of one of the bones of the hand that forms the knuckles, often caused by punching a hard object with a closed fist.

8. Colles' fracture (English) - Fracture de Colles (French) - Fractura de Colles (Spanish) - Colles-Fraktur (German) - Перелом Коллеса (Russian) - 科利斯骨折 (Kē lì sī gǔzhé) (Mandarin)

   - Definition: A fracture of the distal radius bone in the forearm, typically resulting from a fall onto an outstretched hand.

9. Bennett's fracture (English) - Fracture de Bennett (French) - Fractura de Bennett (Spanish) - Bennett-Fraktur (German) - Перелом Беннета (Russian) - 本内特骨折 (Běn nèi tè gǔzhé) (Mandarin)

   - Definition: A fracture of the base of the first metacarpal bone in the thumb.

10. Segond fracture (English) - Fracture de Segond (French) - Fractura de Segond (Spanish) - Segond-Fraktur (German) - Перелом Сегонда (Russian) - 塞冈德骨折 (Sāi gāng dé gǔzhé) (Mandarin)

    - Definition: A specific type of avulsion fracture involving the lateral tibial plateau, often associated with anterior cruciate ligament (ACL) injuries.

11. Hangman's fracture (English) - Fracture du bourreau (French) -

Fractura del verdugo (Spanish) - Henkersfraktur (German) - Повесившегося перелом (Russian) - 绞刑手骨折 (Jiǎoxíng shǒu gǔzhé) (Mandarin)

- Definition: A fracture of the pedicles or pars interarticularis of the second cervical vertebra (C2), typically caused by hyperextension of the neck.

12. Pott's fracture (English) - Fracture de Pott (French) - Fractura de Pott (Spanish) - Pott-Fraktur (German) - Перелом Потта (Russian) - 泊特骨折 (Bó tè gǔzhé) (Mandarin)

- Definition: A fracture of the lower end of the fibula bone in the leg, often associated with a fracture of the lower end of the tibia or dislocation of the ankle joint.

13. Galeazzi fracture (English) - Fracture de Galeazzi (French) - Fractura de Galeazzi (Spanish) - Galeazzi-Fraktur (German) - Перелом Галеаци (Russian) - 盖莱亚骨折 (Gài lái yà gǔzhé) (Mandarin)

- Definition: A fracture of the radius bone in the forearm, often accompanied by dislocation of the distal radioulnar joint.

14. Monteggia fracture (English) - Fracture de Monteggia (French) - Fractura de Monteggia (Spanish) - Monteggia-Fraktur (German) - Перелом Монтеггии (Russian) - 蒙特吉亚骨折 (Mēngtè jíyà gǔzhé) (Mandarin)

- Definition: A fracture of the ulna bone in the forearm, accompanied by dislocation of the radial head.

15. Lisfranc fracture (English) - Fracture de Lisfranc (French) - Fractura de Lisfranc (Spanish) - Lisfranc-Fraktur (German) - Перелом Лисфранка (Russian) - 里斯方骨折 (Lǐ sī fāng gǔzhé) (Mandarin)

- Definition: A fracture or dislocation involving the tarsometatarsal joints in the middle of the foot.

16. Smith's fracture (English) - Fracture de Smith (French) - Fractura de Smith (Spanish) - Smith-Fraktur (German) - Перелом Смита (Russian) - 史密斯骨折 (Shǐ mì sī gǔzhé) (Mandarin)

   - Definition: A fracture of the distal radius with volar displacement of the distal fragment, often resulting from a fall onto a flexed wrist.

17. Barton's fracture (English) - Fracture de Barton (French) - Fractura de Barton (Spanish) - Barton-Fraktur (German) - Перелом Бартона (Russian) - 巴顿骨折 (Bā dùn gǔzhé) (Mandarin)

   - Definition: A fracture of the distal radius with dislocation of the radiocarpal joint, typically occurring as a result of high-energy trauma.

18. Boxer's fracture (English) - Fracture du boxeur (French) - Fractura del boxeador (Spanish) - Boxerfraktur (German) - Перелом боксера (Russian) - 拳击手骨折 (Quánjí shǒu gǔzhé) (Mandarin)

   - Definition: A fracture of one of the bones of the hand that forms the knuckles, often caused by punching a hard object with a closed fist.

19. Hangman's fracture (English) - Fracture du bourreau (French) - Fractura del verdugo (Spanish) - Henkersfraktur (German) - Повесившегося перелом (Russian) - 绞刑手骨折 (Jiǎoxíng shǒu gǔzhé) (Mandarin)

   - Definition: A fracture of the pedicles or pars interarticularis of the second cervical vertebra (C2), typically caused by hyperextension of the neck.

20. Colles' fracture (English) - Fracture de Colles (French) - Fractura de Colles (Spanish) - Colles-Fraktur (German) - Перелом Коллеса (Russian) - 科利斯骨折 (Kē lì sī gǔzhé) (Mandarin)

   - Definition: A fracture of the distal radius bone in the forearm, typically resulting from a fall onto an outstretched hand.

21. Galeazzi fracture (English) - Fracture de Galeazzi (French) - Fractura de Galeazzi (Spanish) - Galeazzi-Fraktur (German) -

Перелом Галеаци (Russian) - 盖莱亚骨折 (Gài lái yà gǔzhé) (Mandarin)

- Definition: A fracture of the radius bone in the forearm, often accompanied by dislocation of the distal radioulnar joint.

22. Monteggia fracture (English) - Fracture de Monteggia (French) - Fractura de Monteggia (Spanish) - Monteggia-Fraktur (German) - Перелом Монтеггии (Russian) - 蒙特吉亚骨折 (Mēngtè jíyà gǔzhé) (Mandarin)

- Definition: A fracture of the ulna bone in the forearm, accompanied by dislocation of the radial head.

23. Lisfranc fracture (English) - Fracture de Lisfranc (French) - Fractura de Lisfranc (Spanish) - Lisfranc-Fraktur (German) - Перелом Лисфранка (Russian) - 里斯方骨折 (Lǐ sī fāng gǔzhé) (Mandarin)

- Definition: A fracture or dislocation involving the tarsometatarsal joints in the middle of the foot.

24. Triplane fracture (English) - Fracture triplane (French) - Fractura triplanar (Spanish) - Dreiflächenfraktur (German) - Трехповерхностный перелом (Russian) - 三面骨折 (Sān miàn gǔzhé) (Mandarin)

- Definition: A fracture that involves three distinct planes of bone, commonly seen in the distal tibia in adolescents.

25. Maisonneuve fracture (English) - Fracture de Maisonneuve (French) - Fractura de Maisonneuve (Spanish) - Maisonneuve-Fraktur (German) - Перелом Мезонёва (Russian) - 梅松涅夫骨折 (Méi sōng niè fū gǔzhé) (Mandarin)

- Definition: A fracture of the proximal third of the fibula with disruption of the syndesmosis, often associated with a spiral fracture of the distal third of the fibula or medial malleolus.

26. Salter-Harris fracture (English) - Fracture de Salter-Harris

(French) - Fractura de Salter-Harris (Spanish) - Salter-Harris-Fraktur (German) - Перелом Солтера-Харриса (Russian) - 萨尔特-哈里斯骨折 (Sà'ěrtè - hā lǐ sī gǔzhé) (Mandarin)

- Definition: A fracture involving the growth plate (physis) of a bone in children and adolescents, classified into different types based on the extent of the injury to the growth plate.

27. Barton's fracture (English) - Fracture de Barton (French) - Fractura de Barton (Spanish) - Barton-Fraktur (German) - Перелом Бартона (Russian) - 巴顿骨折 (Bā dùn gǔzhé) (Mandarin)

- Definition: A fracture of the distal radius with dislocation of the radiocarpal joint, typically occurring as a result of high-energy trauma.

28. Bennett's fracture (English) - Fracture de Bennett (French) - Fractura de Bennett (Spanish) - Bennett-Fraktur (German) - Перелом Беннета (Russian) - 本内特骨折 (Běn nèi tè gǔzhé) (Mandarin)

- Definition: A fracture of the base of the first metacarpal bone in the thumb.

29. Toddler's fracture (English) - Fracture du jeune enfant (French) - Fractura del niño pequeño (Spanish) - Kleinkindfraktur (German) - Перелом у маленького ребенка (Russian) - 幼儿骨折 (Yòu'ér gǔzhé) (Mandarin)

- Definition: A spiral fracture of the tibia in young children, often caused by minor trauma such as a fall while learning to walk.

30. March fracture (English) - Fracture de fatigue (French) - Fractura por estrés (Spanish) - Marschfraktur (German) - Усталостный перелом (Russian) - 行军骨折 (Xíngjūn gǔzhé) (Mandarin)

- Definition: A stress fracture of the metatarsal bones in the foot, typically seen in individuals engaged in repetitive activities like running or marching.

31. Pathological fracture (English) - Fracture pathologique (French) - Fractura patológica (Spanish) - Pathologischer Bruch (German) -

Патологический перелом (Russian) - 病理性骨折 (Bìnglǐ xìng gǔzhé) (Mandarin)

- Definition: A fracture occurring in a bone weakened by a pre-existing condition, such as osteoporosis, infection, or tumor.

32. Stress fracture (English) - Fracture de stress (French) - Fractura por estrés (Spanish) - Ermüdungsbruch (German) - Перелом от нагрузок (Russian) - 应力性骨折 (Yìnglì xìng gǔzhé) (Mandarin)

- Definition: A small crack or severe bruising within a bone due to repetitive application of force, often seen in athletes or military personnel.

33. Boxer's knuckle (English) - Nodule du boxeur (French) - Nudillo del boxeador (Spanish) - Boxerfaust (German) - Костный узел боксера (Russian) - 拳击手拳头 (Quánjí shǒu quántóu) (Mandarin)

- Definition: A type of metacarpal fracture typically affecting the fifth metacarpal bone, also known as a metacarpal neck fracture or a brawler's fracture.

34. Colles' fracture (English) - Fracture de Colles (French) - Fractura de Colles (Spanish) - Colles-Fraktur (German) - Перелом Коллеса (Russian) - 科利斯骨折 (Kē lì sī gǔzhé) (Mandarin)

- Definition: A fracture of the distal radius bone in the forearm, typically resulting from a fall onto an outstretched hand.

35. Galeazzi fracture (English) - Fracture de Galeazzi (French) - Fractura de Galeazzi (Spanish) - Galeazzi-Fraktur (German) - Перелом Галеаци (Russian) - 盖

36. Butterfly fracture (English) - Fracture en ailes de papillon (French) - Fractura en mariposa (Spanish) - Schmetterlingsfraktur (German) - Фрактура бабочки (Russian) - 蝴蝶骨折 (Húdié gǔzhé) (Mandarin)

- Definition: A fracture that involves the splitting of a bone into two fragments, resembling the shape of butterfly wings on X-ray imaging.

37. Boxer's fracture (English) - Fracture du boxeur (French) - Fractura del boxeador (Spanish) - Boxerfraktur (German) - Перелом боксера (Russian) - 拳击手骨折 (Quánjí shǒu gǔzhé) (Mandarin)

   - Definition: A fracture of one of the bones of the hand that forms the knuckles, often caused by punching a hard object with a closed fist.

38. Bennett's fracture (English) - Fracture de Bennett (French) - Fractura de Bennett (Spanish) - Bennett-Fraktur (German) - Перелом Беннета (Russian) - 本内特骨折 (Běn nèi tè gǔzhé) (Mandarin)

   - Definition: A fracture of the base of the first metacarpal bone in the thumb.

39. Toddler's fracture (English) - Fracture du jeune enfant (French) - Fractura del niño pequeño (Spanish) - Kleinkindfraktur (German) - Перелом у маленького ребенка (Russian) - 幼儿骨折 (Yòu'ér gǔzhé) (Mandarin)

   - Definition: A spiral fracture of the tibia in young children, often caused by minor trauma such as a fall while learning to walk.

40. March fracture (English) - Fracture de fatigue (French) - Fractura por estrés (Spanish) - Marschfraktur (German) - Усталостный перелом (Russian) - 行军骨折 (Xíngjūn gǔzhé) (Mandarin)

   - Definition: A stress fracture of the metatarsal bones in the foot, typically seen in individuals engaged in repetitive activities like running or marching.

   41. Pathological fracture (English) - Fracture pathologique (French) - Fractura patológica (Spanish) - Pathologischer Bruch (German) - Патологический перелом (Russian) - 病理性骨折 (Bìnglǐ xìng gǔzhé) (Mandarin)

   - Definition: A fracture occurring in a bone weakened by a pre-existing condition, such as osteoporosis, infection, or tumor.

42. Stress fracture (English) - Fracture de stress (French) - Fractura por estrés (Spanish) - Ermüdungsbruch (German) - Перелом от нагрузок (Russian) - 应力性骨折 (Yìnglì xìng gǔzhé) (Mandarin)

   - Definition: A small crack or severe bruising within a bone due to repetitive application of force, often seen in athletes or military personnel.

43. Boxer's knuckle (English) - Nodule du boxeur (French) - Nudillo del boxeador (Spanish) - Boxerfaust (German) - Костный узел боксера (Russian) - 拳击手拳头 (Quánjí shǒu quántóu) (Mandarin)

   - Definition: A type of metacarpal fracture typically affecting the fifth metacarpal bone, also known as a metacarpal neck fracture or a brawler's fracture.

44. Colles' fracture (English) - Fracture de Colles (French) - Fractura de Colles (Spanish) - Colles-Fraktur (German) - Перелом Коллеса (Russian) - 科利斯骨折 (Kē lì sī gǔzhé) (Mandarin)

   - Definition: A fracture of the distal radius bone in the forearm, typically resulting from a fall onto an outstretched hand.

45. Galeazzi fracture (English) - Fracture de Galeazzi (French) - Fractura de Galeazzi (Spanish) - Galeazzi-Fraktur (German) - Перелом Галеаци (Russian) - 盖莱亚骨折 (Gài lái yà gǔzhé) (Mandarin)

   - Definition: A fracture of the radius bone in the forearm, often accompanied by dislocation of the distal radioulnar joint.

46. Monteggia fracture (English) - Fracture de Monteggia (French) - Fractura de Monteggia (Spanish) - Monteggia-Fraktur (German) - Перелом Монтеггии (Russian) - 蒙特吉亚骨折 (Mēngtè jíyà gǔzhé) (Mandarin)

   - Definition: A fracture of the ulna bone in the forearm, accompanied by dislocation of the radial head.

47. Lisfranc fracture (English) - Fracture de Lisfranc (French) -

Fractura de Lisfranc (Spanish) - Lisfranc-Fraktur (German) - Перелом Лисфранка (Russian) - 里斯方骨折 (Lǐ sī fāng gǔzhé) (Mandarin)

- Definition: A fracture or dislocation involving the tarsometatarsal joints in the middle of the foot.

48. Triplane fracture (English) - Fracture triplane (French) - Fractura triplanar (Spanish) - Dreiflächenfraktur (German) - Трехповерхностный перелом (Russian) - 三面骨折 (Sān miàn gǔzhé) (Mandarin)

- Definition: A fracture that involves three distinct planes of bone, commonly seen in the distal tibia in adolescents.

49. Maisonneuve fracture (English) - Fracture de Maisonneuve (French) - Fractura de Maisonneuve (Spanish) - Maisonneuve-Fraktur (German) - Перелом Мезонёва (Russian) - 梅松涅夫骨折 (Méi sōng niè fū gǔzhé) (Mandarin)

- Definition: A fracture of the proximal third of the fibula with disruption of the syndesmosis, often associated with a spiral fracture of the distal third of the fibula or medial malleolus.

50. Salter-Harris fracture (English) - Fracture de Salter-Harris (French) - Fractura de Salter-Harris (Spanish) - Salter-Harris-Fraktur (German) - Перелом Солтера-Харриса (Russian) - 萨尔特-哈里斯骨折 (Sà'ěrtè - hā lǐ sī gǔzhé) (Mandarin)

- Definition: A fracture involving the growth plate (physis) of a bone in children and adolescents, classified into different types based on the extent of the injury to the growth plate.

1. Sprain (English) - Entorse (French) - Esguince (Spanish) - Verstauchung (German) - Растяжение (Russian) - 扭伤 (Niǔshāng) (Mandarin)

- Definition: An injury to a ligament caused by stretching or tearing.

2. Dislocation (English) - Luxation (French) - Luxación (Spanish) - Luxation (German) - Вывих (Russian) - 脱位 (Tuōwèi) (Mandarin)

   - Definition: The displacement of a bone from its normal position within a joint.

3. Subluxation (English) - Subluxation (French) - Subluxación (Spanish) - Subluxation (German) - Подвывих (Russian) - 半脱位 (Bàn tuōwèi) (Mandarin)

   - Definition: Partial dislocation of a joint where the joint surfaces remain in partial contact.

4. Anterior dislocation (English) - Luxation

5. Posterior dislocation (English) - Luxation antérieure (French) - Luxación anterior (Spanish) - Fornerere Luxation (German) - вывих (Russian) - 面置性脱位 (Mian zhì xìng tuōwèi) (Mandarin)

5. Posterior dislocation (English) - Luxation postérieure (French) - Luxación posterior (Spanish) - Hintere Luxation (German) - Задний вывих (Russian) - 后置性脱位 (Hòu zhì xìng tuōwèi) (Mandarin)

   - Definition: Displacement of a bone from its joint position towards the back of the body.

6. Lateral sprain (English) - Entorse latérale (French) - Esguince lateral (Spanish) - Laterales Bandriss (German) - Боковое растяжение (Russian) - 侧面扭伤 (Cèmiàn niǔshāng) (Mandarin)

   - Definition: Sprain affecting the ligaments on the side of a joint.

7. Medial sprain (English) - Entorse médiale (French) - Esguince medial (Spanish) - Mediales Bandriss (German) - Медиальная растяжение (Russian) - 内侧扭伤 (Nèi cè niǔshāng) (Mandarin)

   - Definition: Sprain affecting the ligaments on the inner side of a joint.

8. High ankle sprain (English) - Entorse de la cheville haute (French) - Esguince de tobillo alto (Spanish) - Hochsprunggelenksverstauchung (German) - Высокое растяжение

голеностопа (Russian) - 高踝扭伤 (Gāo huái niǔshāng) (Mandarin)

   - Definition: Sprain involving the ligaments above the ankle joint, such as the syndesmosis ligament.

9. Low ankle sprain (English) - Entorse de la cheville basse (French) - Esguince de tobillo bajo (Spanish) - Niedriger Sprunggelenksverstauchung (German) - Низкое растяжение голеностопа (Russian) - 低踝扭伤 (Dī huái niǔshāng) (Mandarin)

   - Definition: Sprain affecting the ligaments around the ankle joint.

10. Syndesmosis sprain (English) - Entorse de la syndesmose (French) - Esguince de sindesmosis (Spanish) - Syndesmoseverstauchung (German) - Растяжение связок (Russian) - 韧带扭伤 (Rèndài niǔshāng) (Mandarin)

   - Definition: Sprain involving the syndesmosis ligament connecting the tibia and fibula in the lower leg.

3. EYE ONLY HAVE EYES FOR YOU: EYE INJURIES

1. Conjunctivitis (English) - Conjonctivite (French) - Conjuntivitis (Spanish) - Bindehautentzündung (German) - Конъюнктивит (Russian) - 结膜炎 (Jiémó yán) (Mandarin)

   - Definition: Inflammation of the conjunctiva, the thin membrane covering the white part of the eye and lining the eyelids.

2. Cataract (English) - Cataracte (French) - Catarata (Spanish) - Katarakt (German) - Катаракта (Russian) - 白内障 (Báinèizhàng) (Mandarin)

   - Definition: Clouding of the normally clear lens of the eye, leading to decreased vision.

3. Glaucoma (English) - Glaucome (French) - Glaucoma (Spanish) - Glaukom (German) - Глаукома (Russian) - 青光眼 (Qīngguāngyǎn) (Mandarin)

- Definition: A group of eye conditions that damage the optic nerve, often associated with increased pressure in the eye.

4. Retinal detachment (English) - Détachement de la rétine (French) - Desprendimiento de retina (Spanish) - Netzhautablösung (German) - Отслоение сетчатки (Russian) - 视网膜脱落 (Shìwǎngmó tuōluò) (Mandarin)

- Definition: Separation of the retina, the thin layer of tissue at the back of the eye, from its normal position.

5. Macular degeneration (English) - Dégénérescence maculaire (French) - Degeneración macular (Spanish) - Makuladegeneration (German) - Дегенерация макулы (Russian) - 黄斑变性 (Huángbān biàn xìng) (Mandarin)

- Definition: Progressive deterioration of the macula, the central part of the retina, leading to loss of central vision.

6. Strabismus (English) - Strabisme (French) - Estrabismo (Spanish) - Schielen (German) - Страбизм (Russian) - 斜视 (Xiéshì) (Mandarin)

- Definition: Misalignment of the eyes, causing one or both eyes to turn inward, outward, upward, or downward.

7. Corneal abrasion (English) - Abrasion cornéenne (French) - Abrasión corneal (Spanish) - Hornhautabrieb (German) - Поверхностная повреждение роговицы (Russian) - 角膜擦伤 (Jiǎomó cāshāng) (Mandarin)

- Definition: Scratching or injury to the cornea, the clear front surface of the eye.

8. rosaitis (English) - Blépharite (French) - Blefaritis (Spanish) - Blepharitis (German) - Блефарит (Russian) - 睑板腺炎 (Jiǎnbǎn xiànyán) (Mandarin)

- Definition: Inflammation of the eyelids, usually affecting the edges where the eyelashes grow.

9. Ptosis (English) - Ptosis (French) - Ptosis (Spanish) - Ptosis

(German) - Птоз (Russian) - 下垂眼睑 (Xiàchuí yǎnjiǎn) (Mandarin)

   - Definition: Drooping of the upper eyelid, often due to weakness of the muscles that control eyelid movement.

10. Uveitis (English) - Uvéite (French) - Uveítis (Spanish) - Uveitis (German) - Увеит (Russian) - 葡萄膜炎 (Pútáomó yán) (Mandarin)

   - Definition: Inflammation of the uvea, the middle layer of the eye that includes the iris, ciliary body, and choroid.

   11. Diabetic retinopathy (English) - Rétinopathie diabétique (French) - Retinopatía diabética (Spanish) - Diabetische Retinopathie (German) - Диабетическая ретинопатия (Russian) - 糖尿病性视网膜病变 (Tángniàobìng xìng shìwǎngmó bìngbiàn) (Mandarin)

   - Definition: Damage to the blood vessels of the retina caused by diabetes, leading to vision impairment or blindness.

12. Hyphema (English) - Hyphéma (French) - Hifema (Spanish) - Hyphäma (German) - Гифема (Russian) - 前房积血 (Qián fáng jī xiě) (Mandarin)

   - Definition: Accumulation of blood in the anterior chamber of the eye, often as a result of trauma.

13. Hordeolum (English) - Orgelet (French) - Orzuelo (Spanish) - Hordeolum (German) - Чалазион (Russian) - 麦粒肿 (Màilì zhǒng) (Mandarin)

   - Definition: A localized infection or inflammation of the eyelid margin, commonly known as a stye.

14. Keratitis (English) - Kératite (French) - Queratitis (Spanish) - Keratitis (German) - Кератит (Russian) - 角膜炎 (Jiǎomó yán) (Mandarin)

   - Definition: Inflammation of the cornea, often caused by infection, injury, or underlying conditions.

   15. Amblyopia (English) - Amblyopie (French) - Ambliopía

(Spanish) - Amblyopie (German) - Амблиопия (Russian) - 弱视 (Ruòshì) (Mandarin)

- Definition: Reduced vision in one or both eyes due to abnormal visual development during infancy or childhood.

16. Keratoconus (English) - Kératocône (French) - Queratocono (Spanish) - Keratokonus (German) - Кератоконус (Russian) - 角膜圆锥 (Jiǎomó yuánzhuī) (Mandarin)

- Definition: A progressive thinning and bulging of the cornea, resulting in distorted vision.

17. Photophobia (English) - Photophobie (French) - Fotofobia (Spanish) - Photophobie (German) - Фотофобия (Russian) - 光过敏 (Guāng guòmǐn) (Mandarin)

- Definition: Sensitivity to light, causing discomfort or pain in the eyes when exposed to bright light.

18. Pinguecula (English) - Pinguecula (French) - Pinguécula (Spanish) - Pinguékulä (German) - Пингвекула (Russian) - 葡萄肿 (Pútáozhǒng) (Mandarin)

- Definition: A yellowish, noncancerous growth on the conjunctiva, typically located near the cornea.

19. Pterygium (English) - Ptérygion (French) - Pterigión (Spanish) - Pterygium (German) - Птеригий (Russian) - 翼状胬肉 (Yì zhuàng nù ròu) (Mandarin)

- Definition: A fleshy growth on the conjunctiva, extending onto the cornea, often associated with exposure to UV light.

20. Retinitis pigmentosa (English) - Rétinite pigmentaire (French) - Retinitis pigmentaria (Spanish) - Retinitis pigmentosa (German) - Ретинит пигментозный (Russian) - 视网膜色素变性 (Shìwǎngmó sèsù biàn xìng) (Mandarin)

- Definition: A group of genetic disorders that cause progressive degeneration of the retina, leading to vision loss.

4. SHOW ME ON THE DOLLY: SYMPTOMATIC DESCRIPTIONS

Medican interpreters and treating personnel can and should use dolls to help patients express their exact injuries. Here are terms used to describe varieities of Cuts Bruises Abrasions and Bleeding

1. Laceration (English) - Lacération (French) - Laceración (Spanish) - Platzwunde (German) - Разрыв (Russian) - 撕裂伤 (Sīliè shāng) (Mandarin)

   - Definition: A deep cut or tear in the skin or flesh, often caused by a sharp object or trauma.

2. Contusion (English) - Contusion (French) - Contusión (Spanish) - Prellung (German) - Контузия (Russian) - 挫伤 (Cuòshāng) (Mandarin)

   - Definition: A bruise or injury to the soft tissue underneath the skin, usually resulting from a blunt force impact.

3. Abrasion (English) - Abrasion (French) - Abrasión (Spanish) - Schürfwunde (German) - Поверхностное повреждение (Russian) - 擦伤 (Cāshāng) (Mandarin)

   - Definition: A superficial wound in which the outer layers of the skin are scraped away, often caused by friction or rubbing against a rough surface.

4. Hematoma (English) - Hématome (French) - Hematoma (Spanish) - Hämatom (German) - Гематома (Russian) - 血肿 (Xiě zhǒng) (Mandarin)

   - Definition: A localized collection of blood outside the blood vessels, typically caused by trauma or injury, resulting in swelling and discoloration of the skin.

5. Incision (English) - Incision (French) - Incisión (Spanish) - Einschnitt (German) - Разрез (Russian) - 切口 (Qiēkǒu) (Mandarin)

   - Definition: A clean, straight cut made intentionally, often during surgical procedures or medical interventions.

6. Puncture wound (English) - Plaie par perforation (French) - Herida punzante (Spanish) - Stichverletzung (German) - Прокол (Russian) - 刺伤 (Cìshāng) (Mandarin)

   - Definition: A wound caused by a sharp, pointed object piercing the skin, such as a nail, needle, or animal bite.

7. Avulsion (English) - Avulsion (French) - Avulsión (Spanish) - Abriss (German) - Авульсия (Russian) - 撕脱 (Sītuō) (Mandarin)

   - Definition: A severe injury in which a portion of the skin or tissue is torn away or forcibly removed from the body.

8. Ecchymosis (English) - Ecchymose (French) - Equimosis (Spanish) - Bluterguss (German) - Экхимоз (Russian) - 瘀斑 (Yū bān) (Mandarin)

   - Definition: Discoloration of the skin caused by the leakage of blood into the surrounding tissues, typically appearing as a purple or blue bruise.

9. Crush injury (English) - Blessure par écrasement (French) - Lesión por aplastamiento (Spanish) - Quetschung (German) - Травма сдавления (Russian) - 压伤 (Yāshāng) (Mandarin)

   - Definition: Trauma caused by a compressive force applied to the body, resulting in damage to the underlying tissues and organs.

10. Excoriation (English) - Excoriation (French) - Excoriación (Spanish) - Abschürfung (German) - Экссудация (Russian) - 磨破 (Mó pò) (Mandarin)

    - Definition: A superficial injury in which the outer layer of the skin is removed or abraded, often resulting in pain and irritation.

11. Wound dehiscence (English) - Déhiscence de la plaie (French) - Dehiscencia de la herida (Spanish) - Wunddehiszenz (German) - Дефицит раны (Russian) - 伤口裂开 (Shāngkǒu liè kāi) (Mandarin)

    - Definition: Separation or opening of a previously closed surgical incision or wound, often due to poor healing or excessive tension on the wound edges.

12. Hemorrhage (English) - Hémorragie (French) - Hemorragia (Spanish) - Blutung (German) - Кровотечение (Russian) - 出血 (Chūxiě) (Mandarin)

   - Definition: Excessive or profuse bleeding from ruptured blood vessels, arteries, or capillaries, which can be internal or external.

13. Seroma (English) - Sérome (French) - Seroma (Spanish) - Serom (German) - Серома (Russian) - 积液 (Jīyè) (Mandarin)

   - Definition: Accumulation of serous fluid in a surgical site or wound cavity, typically resulting from tissue trauma or postoperative complications.

14. Ecchymotic hemorrhage (English) - Hémorragie ecchymotique (French) - Hemorragia equimótica (Spanish) - Ekchymotische Blutung (German) - Экхимозное кровоизлияние (Russian) - 瘀血性出血 (Yūxiě xìng chūxiě) (Mandarin)

   - Definition: Bleeding characterized by the formation of ecchymosis or bruising due to the escape of blood into the surrounding tissues.

15. Crush syndrome (English) - Syndrome de l'écrasement (French) - Síndrome de aplastamiento (Spanish) - Crush-Syndrom (German) - Синдром сдавления (Russian) - 压迫综合征 (Yāpò zōnghézhēng) (Mandarin)

   - Definition: Systemic complications resulting from prolonged compression or crushing of skeletal muscle tissue, leading to the release of toxins and electrolyte imbalances.

16. Penetrating trauma (English) - Traumatisme pénétrant (French) - Trauma penetrante (Spanish) - Durchdringende Verletzung (German) - Проникающая травма (Russian) - 穿透性创伤 (Chuāntòu xìng chuāngshāng) (Mandarin)

   - Definition: Injury caused by the penetration of an object or projectile through the skin and underlying tissues, often resulting in deep wounds and internal damage.

17. Hypovolemic shock (English) - Choc hypovolémique (French) - Shock hipovolémico (Spanish) - Hypovolämischer Schock (German) - Гиповолемический шок (Russian) - 低容量性休克 (Dī róngliàng xìng xiūkè) (Mandarin)

  - Definition: Shock state resulting from severe blood loss or inadequate fluid volume in the circulatory system, leading to decreased tissue perfusion and organ dysfunction.

18. Hemostasis (English) - Hémostase (French) - Hemostasis (Spanish) - Hämostase (German) - Гемостаз (Russian) - 止血 (Zhǐxiě) (Mandarin)

  - Definition: The physiological process of stopping bleeding, typically through vasoconstriction, platelet aggregation, and coagulation cascade activation.

19. Oozing (English) - Exsudation (French) - Exudación (Spanish) - Fließen (German) - Выделение (Russian) - 渗出 (Shènchū) (Mandarin)

  - Definition: Slow, continuous leakage or seepage of blood or other fluids from a wound or injured tissue, often indicative of incomplete hemostasis or poor wound healing.

20. Wound infection (English) - Infection de la plaie (French) - Infección de la herida (Spanish) - Wundinfektion (German) - Инфекция раны (Russian) - 伤口感染 (Shāngkǒu gǎnrǎn) (Mandarin)

  - Definition: Invasion and multiplication of microorganisms within a wound or injured tissue, leading to localized or systemic inflammatory response and impaired healing.

21. Venous bleeding (English) - Saignement veineux (French) - Sangrado venoso (Spanish) - Venöse Blutung (German) - Венозное кровотечение (Russian) - 静脉出血 (Jìngmài chūxiě) (Mandarin)

  - Definition: Bleeding from a vein, characterized by a steady flow of dark red blood, which may be difficult to control without proper medical intervention.

22. Arterial bleeding (English) - Saignement artériel (French) - Sangrado arterial (Spanish) - Arterielle Blutung (German) - Артериальное кровотечение (Russian) - 动脉出血 (Dòngmài chūxiě) (Mandarin)

- Definition: Bleeding from an artery, characterized by spurting or pulsating flow of bright red blood, which can be life-threatening if not promptly controlled.

23. Capillary bleeding (English) - Saignement capillaire (French) - Sangrado capilar (Spanish) - Kapillarblutung (German) - Капиллярное кровотечение (Russian) - 毛细血管出血 (Máoxì xuèguǎn chūxiě) (Mandarin)

- Definition: Bleeding from the smallest blood vessels called capillaries, typically resulting in slow oozing of blood, commonly seen in superficial wounds and abrasions.

24. Hemarthrosis (English) - Hémarthrose (French) - Hemartrosis (Spanish) - Hämarthrose (German) - Гемартроз (Russian) - 关节血肿 (Guānjié xuèzhǒng) (Mandarin)

- Definition: Bleeding into a joint space, often resulting from trauma or hemophilia, causing swelling, pain, and limited range of motion in the affected joint.

25. Hemangioma (English) - Hémangiome (French) - Hemangioma (Spanish) - Hämangiom (German) - Гемангиома (Russian) - 血管瘤 (Xuèguǎn liú) (Mandarin)

- Definition: A benign tumor or abnormal growth of blood vessels, often appearing as a red or purple birthmark on the skin.

26. Hemophilia (English) - Hémophilie (French) - Hemofilia (Spanish) - Hämophilie (German) - Гемофилия (Russian) - 血友病 (Xuèyǒu bìng) (Mandarin)

- Definition: A genetic disorder characterized by deficiency or dysfunction of clotting factors in the blood, leading to prolonged bleeding and easy bruising.

27. Purpura (English) - Purpura (French) - Púrpura (Spanish) - Purpura (German) - Пурпура (Russian) - 紫癜 (Zǐdiàn) (Mandarin)

   - Definition: A condition characterized by the appearance of purple or red discoloration of the skin or mucous membranes due to bleeding underneath the skin.

28. Thrombocytopenia (English) - Thrombopénie (French) - Trombocitopenia (Spanish) - Thrombozytopenie (German) - Тромбоцитопения (Russian) - 血小板减少症 (Xiěxiǎobǎn jiǎnshǎo zhèng) (Mandarin)

   - Definition: A condition characterized by a deficiency of platelets in the blood, resulting in impaired blood clotting and increased risk of bleeding.

29. Petechiae (English) - Pétéchies (French) - Petequias (Spanish) - Petechien (German) - Петехии (Russian) - 紫癜点 (Zǐdiàndiǎn) (Mandarin)

   - Definition: Small, pinpoint-sized red or purple spots on the skin or mucous membranes caused by bleeding beneath the surface due to capillary rupture.

30. Disseminated intravascular coagulation (DIC) (English) - Coagulation intravasculaire disséminée (CIVD) (French) - Coagulación intravascular diseminada (CID) (Spanish) - Disseminierte intravasale Gerinnung (DIC) (German) - Диссеминированное внутрисосудистое свертывание (ДВСС) (Russian) - 弥散性血管内凝血 (Mí sàn xìng xuèguǎn nèi níngxiě) (Mandarin)

   - Definition: A complex disorder characterized by widespread activation of blood clotting throughout the body, leading to both excessive clot formation and bleeding tendencies.

   31. Platelet aggregation (English) - Agrégation plaquettaire (French) - Agregación plaquetaria (Spanish) - Thrombozytenaggregation (German) - Агрегация тромбоцитов (Russian) - 血小板聚集 (Xiěxiǎobǎn jùjí) (Mandarin)

   - Definition: The process by which platelets in the blood adhere to each other, forming a platelet plug at the site of vascular injury to initiate hemostasis.

32. Fibrinolysis (English) - Fibrinolyse (French) - Fibrinólisis (Spanish) - Fibrinolyse (German) - Фибринолиз (Russian) - 纤溶 (Xiān róng) (Mandarin)

   - Definition: The process of breaking down fibrin, the protein that forms blood clots, through the action of enzymes called plasmin, to dissolve clots and prevent excessive clot formation.

33. Hematocrit (English) - Hématocrite (French) - Hematócrito (Spanish) - Hämatokrit (German) - Гематокрит (Russian) - 红细胞比容 (Hóng xìbāo bǐ róng) (Mandarin)

   - Definition: The proportion of red blood cells in the total blood volume, expressed as a percentage, which is an indicator of the blood's oxygen-carrying capacity and viscosity.

34. Coagulopathy (English) - Coagulopathie (French) - Coagulopatía (Spanish) - Koagulopathie (German) - Коагулопатия (Russian) - 凝血功能障碍 (Níngxiě gōngnéng zhàng'ài) (Mandarin)

   - Definition: A disorder of blood coagulation characterized by abnormalities in the clotting process, leading to either excessive bleeding or clot formation.

35. Hemangiectomy (English) - Hémangiectomie (French) - Hemangiectomía (Spanish) - Hämangiektomie (German) - Гемангиэктомия (Russian) - 血管切除术 (Xiěguǎn qiēchú shù) (Mandarin)

   - Definition: Surgical removal or excision of a hemangioma, a benign tumor composed of abnormal blood vessels, to alleviate symptoms or prevent complications.

36. Venipuncture (English) - Ponction veineuse (French) - Punción venosa (Spanish) - Venenpunktion (German) - Венепункция (Russian) - 静脉穿刺 (Jìngmài chuānchī) (Mandarin)

   - Definition: The process of puncturing a vein with a needle to obtain a blood sample for diagnostic testing or medical procedures.

37. Hemopericardium (English) - Hémopéricarde (French) - Hemopericardio (Spanish) - Hämoperikard (German) - Гемоперикард (Russian) - 血性心包积液 (Xiě xìng xīnbāo jīyè) (Mandarin)

   - Definition: Accumulation of blood in the pericardial sac surrounding the heart, often resulting from cardiac trauma, rupture, or bleeding disorders.

38. Hematuria (English) - Hématurie (French) - Hematuria (Spanish) - Hämaturie (German) - Гематурия (Russian) - 血尿 (Xiě niào) (Mandarin)

   - Definition: Presence of blood in the urine, which may indicate underlying urinary tract infections, kidney stones, or kidney disease.

39. Hematoma evacuation (English) - Évacuation d'hématome (French) - Evacuación de hematoma (Spanish) - Hämatomevakuierung (German) - Эвакуация гематомы (Russian) - 血肿清除 (Xiě zhǒng qīngchú) (Mandarin)

   - Definition: Surgical drainage or removal of a hematoma, a localized collection of blood outside the blood vessels, to relieve pressure and prevent complications.

40. Hemophiliac bleed (English) - Saignement hémophile (French) - Sangrado hemofílico (Spanish) - Blutung bei Hämophilie (German) - Кровотечение у гемофилика (Russian) - 血友病出血 (Xiěyǒu bìng chu xiě) (Mandarin)

41. Ecchymosis (English) - Ecchymose (French) - Equimosis (Spanish) - Bluterguss (German) - Экхимоз (Russian) - 瘀斑 (Yū bān) (Mandarin)

   - Definition: A discoloration of the skin resulting from bleeding underneath, typically due to bruising or broken blood vessels.

42. Venous stasis ulcer (English) - Ulcère de stase veineuse (French) - Úlcera por estasis venosa (Spanish) - Venöses Stauungsgeschwür (German) - Венозная стаза (Russian) - 静脉淤血性溃疡 (Jìngmài yūxiě xìng kuìyáng) (Mandarin)

- Definition: An open sore on the leg or ankle due to poor blood circulation, often associated with venous insufficiency or varicose veins.

43. Subcutaneous hematoma (English) - Hématome sous-cutané (French) - Hematoma subcutáneo (Spanish) - Subkutanes Hämatom (German) - Подкожное гематома (Russian) - 皮下血肿 (Píxià xuězhǒng) (Mandarin)

- Definition: A collection of blood under the skin but above the muscle layer, typically caused by trauma or injury.

44. Hematemesis (English) - Hématémèse (French) - Hematemesis (Spanish) - Hämatemesis (German) - Гематемез (Russian) - 呕血 (Ǒu xiě) (Mandarin)

- Definition: Vomiting of blood, often due to gastrointestinal bleeding from conditions such as peptic ulcers, esophageal varices, or gastritis.

45. Arterial thrombosis (English) - Thrombose artérielle (French) - Trombosis arterial (Spanish) - Arterielle Thrombose (German) - Артериальная тромбоз (Russian) - 动脉血栓 (Dòngmài xuèsuān) (Mandarin)

- Definition: Formation of a blood clot within an artery, leading to reduced blood flow and potentially causing tissue damage or organ dysfunction.

46. Disseminated intravascular coagulation (DIC) (English) - Coagulation intravasculaire disséminée (CIVD) (French) - Coagulación intravascular diseminada (CID) (Spanish) - Disseminierte intravasale Gerinnung (DIC) (German) - Диссеминированное внутрисосудистое свертывание (ДВСС) (Russian) - 弥散性血管内凝血 (Mí sàn xìng xuèguǎn nèi níngxiě) (Mandarin)

- Definition: A complex disorder characterized by widespread activation of blood clotting throughout the body, leading to both excessive clot formation and bleeding tendencies.

47. Hemorrhagic stroke (English) - AVC hémorragique (French) -

Accidente cerebrovascular hemorrágico (Spanish) - Hämorrhagischer Schlaganfall (German) - Геморрагический инсульт (Russian) - 出血性脑卒中 (Chūxiě xìng nǎo zúzhòng) (Mandarin)

   - Definition: Stroke caused by the rupture of a blood vessel in the brain, leading to bleeding into the surrounding tissues and neurological deficits.

48. Hematologic malignancy (English) - Malignité hématologique (French) - Malignidad hematológica (Spanish) - Hämatologische Malignität (German) - Гематологическая опухоль (Russian) - 血液恶性肿瘤 (Xiěyè èxìng zhòngliú) (Mandarin)

   - Definition: Cancer that originates in the blood-forming tissues, such as the bone marrow or lymphatic system, leading to abnormal blood cell production and function.

49. Hemorrhoidal bleeding (English) - Saignement hémorroïdaire (French) - Sangrado hemorroidal (Spanish) - Hämorrhoidenblutung (German) - Геморроидальное кровотечение (Russian) - 痔疮出血 (Zhìchuāng chūxiě) (Mandarin)

   - Definition: Bleeding from swollen or inflamed blood vessels in the rectum or anus, known as hemorrhoids, often resulting from straining during bowel movements or constipation.

50. Hemothorax (English) - Hémothorax (French) - Hemothorax (Spanish) - Hämothorax (German) - Гемоторакс (Russian) - 血气胸 (Xiěqì xiōng) (Mandarin)

   - Definition: Accumulation of blood in the pleural cavity surrounding the lungs, typically caused by chest trauma or injury to blood vessels within the chest cavity.

51. Hemoptysis (English) - Hémoptyse (French) - Hemoptisis (Spanish) - Hämoptoe (German) - Гемоптоз (Russian) - 咳血 (Kéxiě) (Mandarin)

   - Definition: Coughing up blood or blood-stained sputum from the respiratory tract, often associated with conditions such as pneumonia, bronchitis, or lung cancer.

52. Factor VIII deficiency (English) - Déficit en facteur VIII (French) - Deficiencia de factor VIII (Spanish) - Faktor-VIII-Mangel (German) - Недостаточность фактора VIII (Russian) - 八号凝血因子缺乏 (Bā hào níngxuè yīnzǐ quēfá) (Mandarin)

   - Definition: Hemophilia A, a hereditary bleeding disorder caused by deficiency or dysfunction of clotting factor VIII, leading to prolonged bleeding and easy bruising.

53. Splenic rupture (English) - Rupture splénique (French) - Ruptura esplénica (Spanish) - Milzruptur (German) - Разрыв селезенки (Russian) - 脾脏破裂 (Pí zàng pòliè) (Mandarin)

   - Definition: Tear or rupture of the spleen, often resulting from trauma to the abdomen, leading to internal bleeding and potential life-threatening complications.

54. Petechial rash (English) - Exanthème pétéchial (French) - Rash petequial (Spanish) - Petechiale Hautausschlag (German) - Петехиальная сыпь (Russian) - 瘀点疹 (Yū diǎn zhěn) (Mandarin)

   - Definition: Small, red or purple spots on the skin caused by bleeding under the skin's surface, often associated with conditions such as meningococcal sepsis or thrombocytopenia.

55. Hemodialysis (English) - Hémodialyse (French) - Hemodiálisis (Spanish) - Hämodialyse (German) - Гемодиализ (Russian) - 血液透析 (Xiěyè tòuxī) (Mandarin)

   - Definition: Medical procedure to remove waste products and excess fluid from the blood when the kidneys are unable to perform their filtration function properly.

56. Intracranial hemorrhage (English) - Hémorragie intracrânienne (French) - Hemorragia intracraneal (Spanish) - Intrakranielle Blutung (German) - Внутричерепное кровоизлияние (Russian) - 颅内出血 (Lú nèi chūxiě) (Mandarin)

   - Definition: Bleeding that occurs within the skull or brain, potentially causing increased intracranial pressure and neurological deficits.

57. Blood transfusion (English) - Transfusion sanguine (French) - Transfusión de sangre (Spanish) - Bluttransfusion (German) - Переливание крови (Russian) - 输血 (Shūxiě) (Mandarin)

   - Definition: The process of transferring blood or blood components from one person (donor) to another (recipient) to replace lost blood volume or treat specific medical conditions.

58. Hematologic disorder (English) - Trouble hématologique (French) - Trastorno hematológico (Spanish) - Hämatologische Störung (German) - Гематологическое расстройство (Russian) - 血液病 (Xiěyè bìng) (Mandarin)

   - Definition: A medical condition affecting the blood and blood-forming tissues, such as anemia, leukemia, or thrombocytopenia.

59. Thrombophlebitis (English) - Thrombophlébite (French) - Tromboflebitis (Spanish) - Thrombophlebitis (German) - Тромбофлебит (Russian) - 静脉炎 (Jìngmài yán) (Mandarin)

   - Definition: Inflammation of a vein with associated blood clot formation, typically causing pain, swelling, and redness along the affected vein.

60. Erythrocyte sedimentation rate (ESR) (English) - Vitesse de sédimentation (VS) (French) - Velocidad de sedimentación (VSG) (Spanish) - Erythrozytensedimentationsrate (ESR) (German) - Скорость оседания эритроцитов (СОЭ) (Russian) - 红细胞沉降率 (Hóng xìbāo chénjiàng lǜ) (Mandarin)

   - Definition: A blood test that measures the rate at which red blood cells settle at the bottom of a tube, often used as a non-specific indicator of inflammation or infection in the body.

5. SICK BURN! BURNS SCALDING AND BLISTERING

1. First-degree burn (English) - Brûlure du premier degré (French) - Quemadura de primer grado (Spanish) - Verbrennung ersten Grades (German) - Ожог первой степени (Russian) - 一度烧伤 (Yī dù shāoshāng) (Mandarin)

- Definition: A minor burn affecting only the outer layer of the skin, characterized by redness, pain, and mild swelling.

2. Second-degree burn (English) - Brûlure du deuxième degré (French) - Quemadura de segundo grado (Spanish) - Verbrennung zweiten Grades (German) - Ожог второй степени (Russian) - 二度烧伤 (Èr dù shāoshāng) (Mandarin)

   - Definition: A burn that affects the outer layer of skin (epidermis) and extends into the dermis, causing pain, redness, swelling, and blistering.

3. Third-degree burn (English) - Brûlure du troisième degré (French) - Quemadura de tercer grado (Spanish) - Verbrennung dritten Grades (German) - Ожог третьей степени (Russian) - 三度烧伤 (Sān dù shāoshāng) (Mandarin)

   - Definition: A severe burn that damages all layers of the skin and underlying tissues, characterized by a charred appearance, numbness, and potential loss of sensation.

4. Thermal burn (English) - Brûlure thermique (French) - Quemadura térmica (Spanish) - Thermische Verbrennung (German) - Термический ожог (Russian) - 热烧伤 (Rè shāoshāng) (Mandarin)

   - Definition: A burn caused by exposure to heat, such as flames, hot objects, or scalding liquids.

5. Chemical burn (English) - Brûlure chimique (French) - Quemadura química (Spanish) - Chemische Verbrennung (German) - Химический ожог (Russian) - 化学烧伤 (Huàxué shāoshāng) (Mandarin)

   - Definition: A burn caused by exposure to corrosive substances, such as acids, alkalis, or strong chemicals, leading to tissue damage and necrosis.

6. Electrical burn (English) - Brûlure électrique (French) - Quemadura eléctrica (Spanish) - Elektrische Verbrennung (German) - Электрический ожог (Russian) - 电烧伤 (Diàn shāoshāng) (Mandarin)

- Definition: A burn resulting from contact with an electrical current, causing tissue damage and internal injuries, often with entry and exit wounds.

7. Flash burn (English) - Brûlure éclair (French) - Quemadura por explosión (Spanish) - Blitzverbrennung (German) - Ожог от вспышки (Russian) - 闪光烧伤 (Shǎnguāng shāoshāng) (Mandarin)

   - Definition: A burn caused by exposure to intense heat or flames for a short duration, often associated with explosions or sudden fires.

8. Radiation burn (English) - Brûlure par radiation (French) - Quemadura por radiación (Spanish) - Strahlenverbrennung (German) - Ожог от радиации (Russian) - 辐射烧伤 (Fúshè shāoshāng) (Mandarin)

   - Definition: A burn resulting from exposure to ionizing radiation, such as X-rays or nuclear radiation, leading to skin damage and radiation sickness.

9. Scald (English) - Brûlure par ébouillantement (French) - Escaldadura (Spanish) - Verbrühung (German) - Ожог кипятком (Russian) - 烫伤 (Tàngshāng) (Mandarin)

   - Definition: A burn caused by hot liquids or steam, often resulting in redness, blistering, and tissue damage.

10. Sunburn (English) - Coup de soleil (French) - Quemadura solar (Spanish) - Sonnenbrand (German) - Солнечный ожог (Russian) - 晒伤 (Shàishāng) (Mandarin)

    - Definition: A burn caused by overexposure to the sun.

11. Frostbite (English) - Gelure (French) - Congelación (Spanish) - Erfrierung (German) - Обморожение (Russian) - 冻伤 (Dòngshāng) (Mandarin)

    - Definition: Tissue damage caused by exposure to extreme cold temperatures, leading to numbness, discoloration, and blistering.

12. Superficial burn (English) - Brûlure superficielle (French) - Quemadura superficial (Spanish) - Oberflächliche Verbrennung (German) - Поверхностный ожог (Russian) - 浅表烧伤 (Qiǎnbiǎo shāoshāng) (Mandarin)

   - Definition: A burn that only affects the outer layer of the skin, characterized by redness, pain, and mild swelling, similar to a first-degree burn.

13. Partial-thickness burn (English) - Brûlure de profondeur partielle (French) - Quemadura de espesor parcial (Spanish) - Teilweise Dicke Verbrennung (German) - Частично толщиной ожог (Russian) - 局部厚度烧伤 (Júbù hòudù shāoshāng) (Mandarin)

   - Definition: A burn that extends through the epidermis and into the dermis, causing blistering, pain, and moderate to severe tissue damage, similar to a second-degree burn.

14. Full-thickness burn (English) - Brûlure de pleine épaisseur (French) - Quemadura de espesor total (Spanish) - Vollständige Dicke Verbrennung (German) - Полное толщиной ожог (Russian) - 全层厚度烧伤 (Quáncéng hòudù shāoshāng) (Mandarin)

   - Definition: A burn that extends through all layers of the skin and may involve underlying tissues, characterized by charring, loss of sensation, and potential need for skin grafting, similar to a third-degree burn.

15. Contact burn (English) - Brûlure par contact (French) - Quemadura por contacto (Spanish) - Kontaktverbrennung (German) - Ожог при контакте (Russian) - 接触烧伤 (Jiēchù shāoshāng) (Mandarin)

   - Definition: A burn caused by direct contact with hot objects or surfaces, resulting in localized tissue damage and blistering.

16. Flame burn (English) - Brûlure par flamme (French) - Quemadura por llamas (Spanish) - Flammenverbrennung (German) - Ожог от огня (Russian) - 火焰烧伤 (Huǒyàn shāoshāng) (Mandarin)

- Definition: A burn caused by exposure to flames or fire, resulting in thermal injury and potential inhalation of toxic gases.

17. Smoke inhalation injury (English) - Lésion par inhalation de fumée (French) - Lesión por inhalación de humo (Spanish) - Rauchinhalationsschaden (German) - Травма от вдыхания дыма (Russian) - 吸入烟雾损伤 (Xīrù yānwù sǔnshāng) (Mandarin)

- Definition: Injury to the respiratory tract caused by inhaling hot gases, chemicals, or particulate matter during a fire, leading to airway irritation, coughing, and potential respiratory compromise.

18. Electrical shock injury (English) - Blessure par électrocution (French) - Lesión por descarga eléctrica (Spanish) - Elektrischer Schock (German) - Электрический удар (Russian) - 电击伤 (Diàn jí shāng) (Mandarin)

- Definition: Injury resulting from direct contact with an electric current, causing tissue damage, cardiac arrhythmias, and potential organ dysfunction.

19. Inhalation burn (English) - Brûlure par inhalation (French) - Quemadura por inhalación (Spanish) - Inhalationsverbrennung (German) - Ожог при вдыхании (Russian) - 吸入烧伤 (Xīrù shāoshāng) (Mandarin)

- Definition: Burn injury affecting the respiratory tract due to inhaling hot gases, smoke, or steam, often associated with respiratory distress and pulmonary complications.

20. Flashover burn (English) - Brûlure par embrasement généralisé (French) - Quemadura por flashover (Spanish) - Flashover-Verbrennung (German) - Ожог от разгара (Russian) - 火灾爆燃烧伤 (Huǒzāi bàorán shāoshāng) (Mandarin)

- Definition: A burn injury caused by a sudden and simultaneous ignition of combustible materials in an enclosed space, resulting in rapid spread of flames and thermal injury to occupants.

21. Chemical splash injury (English) - Blessure par projection chimique (French) - Lesión por salpicadura química (Spanish) - Chemischer Spritzer (German) - Химическое брызги (Russian) -

化学溅伤 (Huàxué jiàn shāng) (Mandarin)

   - Definition: Injury resulting from exposure to chemical substances splashed onto the skin or eyes, causing chemical burns, irritation, and potential tissue damage.

22. Inhalation of toxic fumes (English) - Inhalation de fumées toxiques (French) - Inhalación de humos tóxicos (Spanish) - Einatmen von giftigen Dämpfen (German) - Вдыхание токсичных паров (Russian) - 吸入有毒气体 (Xīrù yǒudú qìtǐ) (Mandarin)

   - Definition: Breathing in harmful gases or vapors produced by burning materials or chemical reactions, leading to respiratory irritation, poisoning, and potential organ damage.

23. Thermal injury to airway (English) - Lésion thermique des voies respiratoires (French) - Lesión térmica de las vías respiratorias (Spanish) - Thermische Verletzung der Atemwege (German) - Термическое повреждение дыхательных путей (Russian) - 呼吸道热损伤 (Hūxī dào rè sǔnshāng) (Mandarin)

   - Definition: Damage to the respiratory passages, including the nose, throat, and lungs, due to inhalation of hot gases or steam, causing airway obstruction and respiratory distress.

24. Frostnip (English) - Gelure superficielle (French) - Congelación superficial (Spanish) - Frostbeulen (German) - Переохлаждение (Russian) - 轻度冻伤 (Qīngdù dòngshāng) (Mandarin)

   - Definition: Mild frostbite affecting the outer layers of the skin, causing numbness, tingling, and redness without permanent tissue damage.

25. Chemical corrosion (English) - Corrosion chimique (French) - Corrosión química (Spanish) - Chemische Korrosion (German) - Химическая коррозия (Russian) - 化学腐蚀 (Huàxué fǔshè) (Mandarin)

   - Definition: Destruction or deterioration of materials, including skin or tissues, caused by chemical reactions with corrosive substances, leading to tissue necrosis and damage.

26. Steam burn (English) - Brûlure à la vapeur (French) - Quemadura por vapor (Spanish) - Dampfverbrennung (German) - Ожог паром (Russian) - 蒸汽烧伤 (Zhēngqì shāoshāng) (Mandarin)

- Definition: Burn injury caused by exposure to hot steam, resulting in tissue damage, blistering, and potential scarring.

27. Inhalation of carbon monoxide (English) - Inhalation de monoxyde de carbone (French) - Inhalación de monóxido de carbono (Spanish) - Einatmen von Kohlenmonoxid (German) - Вдыхание оксида углерода (Russian) - 吸入一氧化碳 (Xīrù yīyǎnghuàtàn) (Mandarin)

- Definition: Breathing in carbon monoxide gas, produced by incomplete combustion of carbon-containing materials, leading to carbon monoxide poisoning and tissue hypoxia.

28. Electrical arc flash burn (English) - Brûlure par arc électrique (French) - Quemadura por arco eléctrico (Spanish) - Elektrische Lichtbogenverbrennung (German) - Ожог от электрической дуги (Russian) - 电弧闪 (Diànhú shǎn) (Mandarin)

- Definition: Burn injury caused by exposure to high-intensity electrical arcs, resulting in thermal injury, tissue damage, and potential vision impairment.

29. Frostbite blister (English) - Ampoule de gelure (French) - Ampolla de congelación (Spanish) - Frostbeulenblase (German) - Пузырь морозного ожога (Russian) - 冻伤水泡 (Dòngshāng shuǐpào) (Mandarin)

- Definition: A fluid-filled blister that forms on the skin after frostbite injury, containing serum or blood, and may lead to tissue necrosis if untreated.

30. Inhalation of smoke particles (English) - Inhalation de particules de fumée (French) - Inhalación de partículas de humo (Spanish) - Einatmen von Rauchpartikeln (German) - Вдыхание частиц дыма (Russian) - 吸入烟雾颗粒 (Xīrù yānwù kēlì) (Mandarin)

- Definition: Breathing in microscopic particles suspended in smoke, leading to respiratory irritation, lung inflammation, and potential long-term respiratory problems.

31. Chemical inhalation injury (English) - Lésion par inhalation de produits chimiques (French) - Lesión por inhalación de sustancias químicas (Spanish) - Inhalation von chemischen Dämpfen (German) - Повреждение при вдыхании химических веществ (Russian) - 化学气体吸入伤 (Huàxué qìtǐ xīrù shāng) (Mandarin)

   - Definition: Injury to the respiratory system caused by inhaling toxic or irritating chemical fumes or gases, leading to airway inflammation, lung damage, and systemic toxicity.

32. Frostbite gangrene (English) - Gangrène de gelure (French) - Gangrena por congelación (Spanish) - Frostbeulen-Gangrän (German) - Гангрена морозного ожога (Russian) - 冻伤坏死 (Dòngshāng huàisǐ) (Mandarin)

   - Definition: Tissue death (gangrene) resulting from severe frostbite injury, characterized by blackened, necrotic tissue and potential need for surgical intervention or amputation.

33. Flame inhalation injury (English) - Lésion par inhalation de flammes (French) - Lesión por inhalación de llamas (Spanish) - Flammeninhalationsschaden (German) - Травма при вдыхании огня (Russian) - 火焰吸入伤 (Huǒyàn xīrù shāng) (Mandarin)

   - Definition: Damage to the respiratory tract caused by inhaling hot gases and flames during a fire, leading to airway burns, lung injury, and potential respiratory failure.

34. Electrical contact burn (English) - Brûlure par contact électrique (French) - Quemadura por contacto eléctrico (Spanish) - Elektrische Kontaktverbrennung (German) - Ожог при контакте с электричеством (Russian) - 电击接触烧伤 (Diàn jí jiēchù shāoshāng) (Mandarin)

   - Definition: Burn injury resulting from direct contact with an electrical source, such as a live wire or electrical appliance, causing tissue damage and potential internal injuries.

35. Chemical exposure rash (English) - Éruption cutanée due à une exposition chimique (French) - Sarpullido por exposición química (Spanish) - Hautausschlag durch chemische Exposition (German) - Сыпь после контакта с химическими веществами (Russian) - 化学物质接触皮疹 (Huàxué wùzhì jiēchù pízhěn) (Mandarin)

  - Definition: Skin rash or irritation caused by exposure to chemical substances, resulting in redness, itching, and inflammation of the skin.

36. Inhalation of caustic fumes (English) - Inhalation de vapeurs caustiques (French) - Inhalación de vapores cáusticos (Spanish) - Einatmen von ätzenden Dämpfen (German) - Вдыхание едких паров (Russian) - 吸入腐蚀性气体 (Xīrù fǔsè xìng qìtǐ) (Mandarin)

  - Definition: Breathing in corrosive or irritant fumes that can cause chemical burns to the respiratory tract, leading to airway injury and pulmonary complications.

37. Flame scorch injury (English) - Lésion par brûlure superficielle (French) - Lesión por quemadura superficial (Spanish) - Flammenversengungsschaden (German) - Повреждение от пламени (Russian) - 火焰烧伤灼伤 (Huǒyàn shāoshāng zhuóshāng) (Mandarin)

  - Definition: Superficial burn injury caused by exposure to flames, resulting in reddened, scorched skin and mild tissue damage.

38. Inhalation of smoke toxins (English) - Inhalation de toxines de fumée (French) - Inhalación de toxinas del humo (Spanish) - Einatmen von Rauchtoxinen (German) - Вдыхание токсинов дыма (Russian) - 吸入烟毒素 (Xīrù yān dúsù) (Mandarin)

  - Definition: Breathing in harmful chemicals and toxins present in smoke, leading to systemic toxicity, respiratory irritation, and potential long-term health effects.

39. Chemical eye splash (English) - Projection chimique dans les yeux (French) - Salpicadura química en los ojos (Spanish) - Chemischer Augenkontakt (German) - Химическое попадание в

глаза (Russian) - 化学物质溅入眼睛 (Huàxué wùzhì jiàn rù yǎnjīng) (Mandarin)

   - Definition: Injury to the eyes caused by exposure to chemical substances, resulting in irritation, redness, and potential corneal damage.

40. Flash fire burn (English) - Brûlure par feu de flash (French) - Quemadura por fuego repentino (Spanish) - Blitzbrandverbrennung (German) - Ожог от вспышки огня (Russian) - 火光烧伤 (Huǒguāng shāoshāng) (Mandarin)

- Definition: Burn injury caused by sudden ignition of combustible materials, leading to rapid spread of flames and thermal injury to the skin.

6. CAN YOU STOMACH THIS? ESOPHAGAL INJURIES

   1. Gastroesophageal reflux disease (GERD) (English) - Reflux gastro-œsophagien (French) - Enfermedad por reflujo gastroesofágico (Spanish) - Gastroösophageale Refluxkrankheit (German) - Болезнь гастроэзофагеального рефлюкса (Russian) - 胃食管反流病 (Wèi shíguǎn fǎnliú bìng) (Mandarin)

   - Definition: A chronic condition where stomach acid regularly flows back into the esophagus, causing irritation and inflammation of the esophageal lining.

2. Peptic ulcer disease (English) - Ulcère gastro-duodénal (French) - Enfermedad ulcerosa péptica (Spanish) - Magengeschwürkrankheit (German) - Язва желудка и двенадцатиперстной кишки (Russian) - 消化性溃疡病 (Xiāohuà xìng kuìyáng bìng) (Mandarin)

   - Definition: A condition characterized by the formation of open sores (ulcers) on the lining of the stomach or duodenum, often caused by infection with Helicobacter pylori bacteria or prolonged use of nonsteroidal anti-inflammatory drugs (NSAIDs).

3. Esophageal stricture (English) - Sténose de l'œsophage (French) - Estenosis esofágica (Spanish) - Ösophagusstenose (German) -

Стеноз пищевода (Russian) - 食管狭窄 (Shíguǎn xiázhǎi) (Mandarin)

- Definition: Narrowing of the esophagus, usually due to scar tissue formation or inflammation, leading to difficulty swallowing and potential food impaction.

4. Gastric perforation (English) - Perforation gastrique (French) - Perforación gástrica (Spanish) - Magenperforation (German) - Желудочное перфорирование (Russian) - 胃穿孔 (Wèi chuānkǒng) (Mandarin)

- Definition: A hole or tear in the wall of the stomach, often caused by peptic ulcers, trauma, or certain medical procedures, leading to leakage of stomach contents into the abdominal cavity.

5. Achalasia (English) - Achalasie (French) - Acalasia (Spanish) - Achalasie (German) - Ахалазия (Russian) - 气管扩张 (Qìguǎn kuòzhǎng) (Mandarin)

- Definition: A disorder of the esophagus where the lower esophageal sphincter fails to relax properly, leading to difficulty swallowing, regurgitation, and chest pain.

6. Dental avulsion (English) - Avulsion dentaire (French) - Avulsión dental (Spanish) - Zahnentfernung (German) - Вырывание зубов (Russian) - 牙齿脱位 (Yáchǐ tuōwèi) (Mandarin)

- Definition: Complete displacement of a tooth from its socket due to trauma or injury, often resulting in bleeding, pain, and potential tooth loss.

7. Oral laceration (English) - Lésion buccale (French) - Laceración oral (Spanish) - Mundschleimhautlaceration (German) - Порез во рту (Russian) - 口腔撕裂伤 (Kǒuqiāng sīliè shāng) (Mandarin)

- Definition: A cut or tear in the oral mucosa or tissues of the mouth, often caused by trauma, dental procedures, or sharp objects, leading to pain and potential infection.

8. Esophageal varices (English) - Varices œsophagiennes (French) - Varices esofágicas (Spanish) - Ösophagusvarizen (German) -

Варикозное расширение пищевода (Russian) - 食管静脉曲张 (Shíguǎn jìngmài qūzhāng) (Mandarin)

   - Definition: Dilated and swollen veins in the esophagus, often caused by liver cirrhosis and portal hypertension, which can lead to gastrointestinal bleeding and life-threatening complications.

9. Dental fracture (English) - Fracture dentaire (French) - Fractura dental (Spanish) - Zahnfraktur (German) - Перелом зуба (Russian) - 牙骨折 (Yá gǔ zhé) (Mandarin)

   - Definition: A break or crack in a tooth, often caused by trauma, biting on hard objects, or dental decay, leading to pain and potential tooth loss.

10. Esophageal cancer (English) - Cancer de l'œsophage (French) - Cáncer de esófago (Spanish) - Ösophaguskarzinom (German) - Рак пищевода (Russian) - 食管癌 (Shíguǎn ái) (Mandarin)

   - Definition: Malignant tumor that develops in the tissues of the esophagus, often associated with smoking, heavy alcohol consumption, and chronic acid reflux, leading to difficulty swallowing, weight loss, and other symptoms.

      11. Gastric ulcer (English) - Ulcère gastrique (French) - Úlcera gástrica (Spanish) - Magengeschwür (German) - Язва желудка (Russian) - 胃溃疡 (Wèi kuìyáng) (Mandarin)

   - Definition: A sore that forms on the inner lining of the stomach, often due to bacterial infection with Helicobacter pylori or prolonged use of nonsteroidal anti-inflammatory drugs (NSAIDs).

12. Esophageal spasm (English) - Spasme œsophagien (French) - Espasmo esofágico (Spanish) - Ösophagusspasmus (German) - Спазм пищевода (Russian) - 食管痉挛 (Shíguǎn jìngluán) (Mandarin)

   - Definition: Involuntary contractions or tightening of the muscles in the esophagus, causing chest pain, difficulty swallowing, and a sensation of food getting stuck.

13. Oral candidiasis (English) - Candidose buccale (French) -

Candidiasis oral (Spanish) - Mundsoor (German) - Оральный кандидоз (Russian) - 口腔念珠菌病 (Kǒuqiāng niànzhūjūn bìng) (Mandarin)

   - Definition: Fungal infection of the mouth caused by Candida yeast, characterized by white patches on the tongue, inner cheeks, and throat, often seen in immunocompromised individuals.

14. Esophageal stricture (English) - Sténose de l'œsophage (French) - Estenosis esofágica (Spanish) - Ösophagusstenose (German) - Стеноз пищевода (Russian) - 食管狭窄 (Shíguǎn xiázhǎi) (Mandarin)

   - Definition: Narrowing of the esophagus, often due to scar tissue formation or inflammation, leading to difficulty swallowing and potential food impaction.

15. Dental abscess (English) - Abcès dentaire (French) - Absceso dental (Spanish) - Zahnabszess (German) - Зубной абсцесс (Russian) - 牙周脓肿 (Yá zhōu nóngzhǒng) (Mandarin)

   - Definition: Collection of pus within the tooth or surrounding tissues, often caused by bacterial infection, leading to severe toothache, swelling, and potential systemic complications.

16. Gastroesophageal junction (English) - Jonction gastro-œsophagienne (French) - Unión gastroesofágica (Spanish) - Magen-Darm-Mündung (German) - Переход желудка и пищевода (Russian) - 胃食管交界 (Wèi shíguǎn jiāojiè) (Mandarin)

   - Definition: The area where the esophagus meets the stomach, responsible for regulating the passage of food and preventing reflux of stomach contents into the esophagus.

17. Dental caries (English) - Carie dentaire (French) - Caries dental (Spanish) - Zahnkaries (German) - Кариес зубов (Russian) - 龋齿 (Qū chǐ) (Mandarin)

   - Definition: Tooth decay caused by bacterial erosion of tooth enamel, leading to cavities, tooth sensitivity, and potential tooth loss if untreated.

18. Esophageal motility disorder (English) - Trouble moteur de l'œsophage (French) - Trastorno de motilidad esofágica (Spanish) - Ösophagusmotilitätsstörung (German) - Расстройство моторики пищевода (Russian) - 食管运动障碍 (Shíguǎn yùndòng zhàng'ài) (Mandarin)

 - Definition: Abnormalities in the coordinated muscle contractions of the esophagus, leading to swallowing difficulties, chest pain, and regurgitation of food or liquids.

19. Oral leukoplakia (English) - Leucoplasie buccale (French) - Leucoplasia oral (Spanish) - Leukoplakie (German) - Лейкоплакия полости рта (Russian) - 口腔白斑病 (Kǒuqiāng báibān bìng) (Mandarin)

 - Definition: Thickened, white patches or lesions that develop on the mucous membranes of the mouth, often associated with tobacco use or chronic irritation, and may indicate a precancerous condition.

20. Esophageal diverticulum (English) - Diverticule de l'œsophage (French) - Divertículo esofágico (Spanish) - Ösophagusdivertikel (German) - Пищеводное грыжа (Russian) - 食管憩室 (Shíguǎn qìshì) (Mandarin)

 - Definition: A pouch or sac that forms in the wall of the esophagus, causing difficulty swallowing, regurgitation, and potential food trapping.

21. Oral thrush (English) - Muguet buccal (French) - Candidiasis oral (Spanish) - Mundsoor (German) - Оральный трихофитоз (Russian) - 口腔念珠菌病 (Kǒuqiāng niànzhūjūn bìng) (Mandarin)

 - Definition: Fungal infection of the mouth caused by Candida yeast, characterized by white patches on the tongue, inner cheeks, and throat, often seen in immunocompromised individuals.

22. Gastroesophageal junction (English) - Jonction gastro-œsophagienne (French) - Unión gastroesofágica (Spanish) - Magen-Darm-Mündung (German) - Переход желудка и пищевода (Russian) - 胃食管交界 (Wèi shíguǎn jiāojiè) (Mandarin)

- Definition: The area where the esophagus meets the stomach, responsible for regulating the passage of food and preventing reflux of stomach contents into the esophagus.

23. Dental caries (English) - Carie dentaire (French) - Caries dental (Spanish) - Zahnkaries (German) - Кариес зубов (Russian) - 龋齿 (Qū chǐ) (Mandarin)

- Definition: Tooth decay caused by bacterial erosion of tooth enamel, leading to cavities, tooth sensitivity, and potential tooth loss if untreated.

24. Esophageal motility disorder (English) - Trouble moteur de l'œsophage (French) - Trastorno de motilidad esofágica (Spanish) - Ösophagusmotilitätsstörung (German) - Расстройство моторики пищевода (Russian) - 食管运动障碍 (Shíguǎn yùndòng zhàng'ài) (Mandarin)

- Definition: Abnormalities in the coordinated muscle contractions of the esophagus, leading to swallowing difficulties, chest pain, and regurgitation of food or liquids.

25. Oral leukoplakia (English) - Leucoplasie buccale (French) - Leucoplasia oral (Spanish) - Leukoplakie (German) - Лейкоплакия полости рта (Russian) - 口腔白斑病 (Kǒuqiāng báibān bìng) (Mandarin)

- Definition: Thickened, white patches or lesions that develop on the mucous membranes of the mouth, often associated with tobacco use or chronic irritation, and may indicate a precancerous condition.

26. Esophageal diverticulum (English) - Diverticule de l'œsophage (French) - Divertículo esofágico (Spanish) - Ösophagusdivertikel (German) - Пищеводное грыжа (Russian) - 食管憩室 (Shíguǎn qìshì) (Mandarin)

- Definition: A pouch or sac that forms in the wall of the esophagus, causing difficulty swallowing, regurgitation, and potential food trapping.

27. Oral submucous fibrosis (English) - Fibrose sous-muqueuse buccale (French) - Fibrosis submucosa oral (Spanish) - Submuköse

orale Fibrose (German) - Оральный субмукозный фиброз (Russian) - 口腔粘膜下纤维增生 (Kǒuqiāng zhānmú xià xiānwéi zēngshēng) (Mandarin)

   - Definition: Chronic, progressive scarring and fibrosis of the oral mucosa, often associated with betel nut chewing and smoking, leading to difficulty in opening the mouth and potential oral cancer.

28. Zenker's diverticulum (English) - Diverticule de Zenker (French) - Divertículo de Zenker (Spanish) - Zenker-Divertikel (German) - Дивертикул Зенкера (Russian) - 钱克尔憩室 (Qián kè ěr qìshì) (Mandarin)

   - Definition: A pouch or sac that forms at the back of the throat, just above the esophagus, leading to difficulty swallowing, regurgitation, and potential aspiration of food or fluids.

29. Oral cancer (English) - Cancer de la bouche (French) - Cáncer oral (Spanish) - Mundkrebs (German) - Рак полости рта (Russian) - 口腔癌 (Kǒuqiāng ái) (Mandarin)

   - Definition: Malignant tumor that develops in the tissues of the mouth, often associated with tobacco use, alcohol consumption, and human papillomavirus (HPV).

30. Esophageal varices (English) - Varices œsophagiennes (French) - Varices esofágicas (Spanish) - Ösophagusvarizen (German) - Варикозное расширение пищевода (Russian) - 食管静脉曲张 (Shíguǎn jìngmài qūzhāng) (Mandarin)

   - Definition: Dilated and swollen veins in the esophagus, often caused by liver cirrhosis and portal hypertension, which can lead to gastrointestinal bleeding and life-threatening complications.

31. Gingivitis (English) - Gingivite (French) - Gingivitis (Spanish) - Gingivitis (German) - Гингивит (Russian) - 牙龈炎 (Yágǔnyán) (Mandarin)

   - Definition: Inflammation of the gums, characterized by redness, swelling, and bleeding, often caused by poor oral hygiene or bacterial infection.

32. Esophageal ring (English) - Anneau œsophagien (French) - Anillo esofágico (Spanish) - Ösophagusring (German) - Кольцо пищевода (Russian) - 食管环 (Shíguǎn huán) (Mandarin)

- Definition: A band or narrowing in the esophagus, often congenital or acquired, leading to difficulty swallowing and potential food impaction.

33. Dental plaque (English) - Plaque dentaire (French) - Placa dental (Spanish) - Zahnbelag (German) - Зубной налет (Russian) - 牙菌斑 (Yá jūnbān) (Mandarin)

- Definition: A sticky film of bacteria that forms on the teeth, leading to tooth decay, gum disease, and bad breath if not removed through regular brushing and flossing.

34. Esophageal ulcer (English) - Ulcère de l'œsophage (French) - Úlcera esofágica (Spanish) - Ösophagusulkus (German) - Язва пищевода (Russian) - 食管溃疡 (Shíguǎn kuìyáng) (Mandarin)

- Definition: A sore or lesion that develops on the lining of the esophagus, often caused by acid reflux, infections, or medications, leading to pain and difficulty swallowing.

35. Oral torus (English) - Torus buccal (French) - Torus oral (Spanish) - Mundtorus (German) - Оральный торус (Russian) - 口腔骨骼肿瘤 (Kǒuqiāng gǔgé zhǒngliú) (Mandarin)

- Definition: Benign bony growth that protrudes from the surface of the jaw or palate, often asymptomatic but may interfere with speech or eating in severe cases.

36. Pharyngitis (English) - Pharyngite (French) - Faringitis (Spanish) - Pharyngitis (German) - Фарингит (Russian) - 咽炎 (Yān yán) (Mandarin)

- Definition: Inflammation of the pharynx (throat), characterized by sore throat, difficulty swallowing, and swollen lymph nodes, often caused by viral or bacterial infections.

37. Dental erosion (English) - Érosion dentaire (French) - Erosión dental (Spanish) - Zahnsubstanzverlust (German) - Эрозия зубов (Russian) - 牙齿磨损 (Yáchǐ mó sǔn) (Mandarin)

   - Definition: Progressive loss of tooth enamel due to acid exposure, often from acidic foods, beverages, or gastric reflux, leading to tooth sensitivity and increased risk of cavities.

38. Barrett's esophagus (English) - Œsophage de Barrett (French) - Esófago de Barrett (Spanish) - Barrett-Ösophagus (German) - Эзофагит Барретта (Russian) - 巴雷特食管 (Bāléitè shíguǎn) (Mandarin)

   - Definition: A condition where the normal cells lining the esophagus are replaced by abnormal cells, often due to chronic acid reflux, increasing the risk of esophageal cancer.

39. Oral herpes (English) - Herpès buccal (French) - Herpes oral (Spanish) - Mundherpes (German) - Герпес полости рта (Russian) - 口唇疱疹 (Kǒuchún páozhěn) (Mandarin)

   - Definition: Viral infection caused by the herpes simplex virus (HSV) affecting the mouth and lips, characterized by painful blisters or cold sores.

40. Esophageal candidiasis (English) - Candidose œsophagienne (French) - Candidiasis esofágica (Spanish) - Ösophagale Candidiasis (German) - Кандид

41. Oral leukoplakia (English) - Leucoplasie buccale (French) - Leucoplasia oral (Spanish) - Leukoplakie (German) - Лейкоплакия полости рта (Russian) - 口腔白斑病 (Kǒuqiāng báibān bìng) (Mandarin)

   - Definition: Thickened, white patches or lesions that develop on the mucous membranes of the mouth, often associated with tobacco use or chronic irritation, and may indicate a precancerous condition.

42. Esophageal diverticulum (English) - Diverticule de l'œsophage (French) - Divertículo esofágico (Spanish) - Ösophagusdivertikel (German) - Пищеводное грыжа (Russian) - 食管憩室 (Shíguǎn

qìshì) (Mandarin)

   - Definition: A pouch or sac that forms in the wall of the esophagus, causing difficulty swallowing, regurgitation, and potential food trapping.

43. Oral submucous fibrosis (English) - Fibrose sous-muqueuse buccale (French) - Fibrosis submucosa oral (Spanish) - Submuköse orale Fibrose (German) - Оральный субмукозный фиброз (Russian) - 口腔粘膜下纤维增生 (Kǒuqiāng zhānmú xià xiānwéi zēngshēng) (Mandarin)

   - Definition: Chronic, progressive scarring and fibrosis of the oral mucosa, often associated with betel nut chewing and smoking, leading to difficulty in opening the mouth and potential oral cancer.

44. Zenker's diverticulum (English) - Diverticule de Zenker (French) - Divertículo de Zenker (Spanish) - Zenker-Divertikel (German) - Дивертикул Зенкера (Russian) - 钱克尔憩室 (Qián kè ěr qìshì) (Mandarin)

   - Definition: A pouch or sac that forms at the back of the throat, just above the esophagus, leading to difficulty swallowing, regurgitation, and potential aspiration of food or fluids.

45. Oral cancer (English) - Cancer de la bouche (French) - Cáncer oral (Spanish) - Mundkrebs (German) - Рак полости рта (Russian) - 口腔癌 (Kǒuqiāng ái) (Mandarin)

   - Definition: Malignant tumor that develops in the tissues of the mouth, often associated with tobacco use, alcohol consumption, and human papillomavirus (HPV).

7. COUGH IT UP! Terms related to symptoms of coughing:

1. Cough (English) - Toux (French) - Tos (Spanish) - Husten (German) - Кашель (Russian) - 咳嗽 (Késou) (Mandarin)

   - Definition: A sudden expulsion of air from the lungs typically accompanied by a distinctive sound, often due to irritation or infection in the respiratory tract.

2. Phlegm (English) - Mucus (French) - Flemas (Spanish) - Schleim (German) - Мокрота (Russian) - 痰 (Tán) (Mandarin)

   - Definition: Thick, sticky secretion produced by the mucous membranes in the respiratory tract, often expelled during coughing.

3. Sore throat (English) - Mal de gorge (French) - Dolor de garganta (Spanish) - Halsschmerzen (German) - Боль в горле (Russian) - 喉咙痛 (Hóulóng tòng) (Mandarin)

   - Definition: Pain or irritation in the throat, often worsened by coughing, swallowing, or talking.

4. Wheezing (English) - Sifflement (French) - Sibilancias (Spanish) - Pfeifen (German) - Хрипы (Russian) - 喘鸣 (Chuǎn míng) (Mandarin)

   - Definition: High-pitched whistling sound made while breathing, often associated with narrowed airways due to inflammation or obstruction.

5. Chest congestion (English) - Congestion thoracique (French) - Congestión torácica (Spanish) - Brustenge (German) - Загрудинная

конгестия (Russian) - 胸部充血 (Xiōngbù chōngxiě) (Mandarin)

- Definition: Feeling of fullness or heaviness in the chest, often accompanied by difficulty breathing, due to the accumulation of mucus or fluid in the lungs.

6. Dry cough (English) - Toux sèche (French) - Tos seca (Spanish) - Trockener Husten (German) - Сухой кашель (Russian) - 干咳 (Gān késou) (Mandarin)

- Definition: Cough that does not produce phlegm or mucus, often caused by irritation or inflammation in the throat or airways.

7. Productive cough (English) - Toux productive (French) - Tos productiva (Spanish) - Produktiver Husten (German) - Продуктивный кашель (Russian) - 有痰咳嗽 (Yǒu tán késou) (Mandarin)

- Definition: Cough that brings up mucus or phlegm from the lungs, often seen in respiratory infections or lung diseases.

8. Irritated throat (English) - Gorge irritée (French) - Garganta irritada (Spanish) - Reizhusten (German) - Раздраженное горло (Russian) - 喉咙痒 (Hóulóng yǎng) (Mandarin)

- Definition: Sensation of discomfort or tickling in the throat, often leading to coughing reflex.

9. Chest pain with cough (English) - Douleur thoracique avec toux (French) - Dolor de pecho con tos (Spanish) - Brustschmerzen beim Husten (German) - Боль в груди при кашле (Russian) - 咳嗽时胸痛 (Késou shí xiōng tòng) (Mandarin)

- Definition: Pain or discomfort in the chest that worsens with coughing, which can be indicative of various respiratory or cardiac conditions.

10. Barking cough (English) - Toux aboyante (French) - Tos perruna (Spanish) - Bellender Husten (German) - Лающий кашель (Russian) - 咳嗽声似狗叫 (Késou shēng sì gǒu jiào) (Mandarin)

- Definition: Harsh, dry cough resembling the sound of a dog's bark, often associated with croup or other upper respiratory infections.

11. Hacking cough (English) - Toux rauque (French) - Tos seca y fuerte (Spanish) - Rauer Husten (German) - Хриплый кашель (Russian) - 干咳 (Gān késou) (Mandarin)

   - Definition: Persistent, forceful cough characterized by repeated, harsh sound, often due to irritation or inflammation in the throat.

12. Tickling in the throat (English) - Chatouillement dans la gorge (French) - Cosquilleo en la garganta (Spanish) - Kratzen im Hals (German) - Щекотание в горле (Russian) - 喉咙痒 (Hóulóng yǎng) (Mandarin)

   - Definition: Sensation of slight irritation or discomfort in the throat, often leading to a reflexive cough to alleviate the sensation.

13. Hoarse voice (English) - Voix rauque (French) - Voz ronca (Spanish) - Heisere Stimme (German) - Хриплый голос (Russian) - 嗓音沙哑 (Sǎng yīn shā yǎ) (Mandarin)

   - Definition: Voice that is rough, raspy, or strained, often due to inflammation or irritation of the vocal cords from coughing or other causes.

14. Rattling in the chest (English) - Râles dans la poitrine (French) - Ruidos en el pecho (Spanish) - Rasseln in der Brust (German) - Хрипы в груди (Russian) - 胸部嘶嘶声 (Xiōngbù sī sī shēng) (Mandarin)

   - Definition: Abnormal sounds heard during breathing, resembling rattling or gurgling, often due to the presence of mucus or fluid in the lungs.

15. Difficulty breathing with cough (English) - Difficulté à respirer avec toux (French) - Dificultad para respirar con tos (Spanish) - Atembeschwerden beim Husten (German) - Затрудненное дыхание при кашле (Russian) - 咳嗽时呼吸困难 (Késou shí hūxī kùnnán) (Mandarin)

   - Definition: Feeling of breathlessness or shortness of breath that worsens with coughing, indicating possible airway obstruction or respiratory distress.

16. Blood in the sputum (English) - Sang dans les crachats (French) - Sangre en el esputo (Spanish) - Blut im Auswurf (German) - Кровь в мокроте (Russian) - 痰中有血 (Tán zhōng yǒu xiě) (Mandarin)

   - Definition: Presence of blood in the mucus or phlegm coughed up from the lungs or airways, which can indicate various respiratory conditions such as bronchitis, pneumonia, or lung cancer.

17. Persistent cough (English) - Toux persistante (French) - Tos persistente (Spanish) - Anhaltender Husten (German) - Постоянный кашель (Russian) - 持续性咳嗽 (Chíxù xìng késou) (Mandarin)

   - Definition: Cough that lasts for an extended period, typically more than two to three weeks, often indicating an underlying chronic condition such as asthma, bronchitis, or gastroesophageal reflux disease (GERD).

18. Coughing fits (English) - Accès de toux (French) - Ataques de tos (Spanish) - Hustenanfälle (German) - Пароксизмальный кашель (Russian) - 咳嗽发作 (Késou fāzuò) (Mandarin)

   - Definition: Episodes of intense or prolonged coughing, often occurring in rapid succession and causing significant discomfort or distress to the patient.

19. Chest tightness (English) - Serrement de poitrine (French) - Opresión en el pecho (Spanish) - Beklemmung in der Brust (German) - Сдавление в груди (Russian) - 胸闷 (Xiōng mèn) (Mandarin)

   - Definition: Feeling of pressure, heaviness, or discomfort in the chest, often associated with coughing and difficulty breathing, indicative of various respiratory or cardiac conditions.

20. Choking sensation (English) - Sensation d'étouffement (French) - Sensación de atragantamiento (Spanish) - Erstickungsgefühl (German) - Ощущение задыхания (Russian) - 感觉窒息 (Gǎnjué zhìxí) (Mandarin)

- Definition: Feeling of obstruction or blockage in the throat or airways, leading to difficulty breathing or coughing, often associated with choking on food or foreign objects, or respiratory conditions such as asthma or chronic obstructive pulmonary disease (COPD).

21. Rib pain with cough (English) - Douleur aux côtes avec toux (French) - Dolor en las costillas con tos (Spanish) - Rippen schmerzen beim Husten (German) - Боль в рёбрах при кашле (Russian) - 咳嗽时肋骨疼痛 (Késou shí lèi gǔ téngtòng) (Mandarin)

- Definition: Pain or discomfort in the ribs that worsens with coughing, which can indicate various conditions such as rib fracture, muscle strain, or pleurisy.

22. Shortness of breath (English) - Essoufflement (French) - Falta de aire (Spanish) - Atemnot (German) - Одышка (Russian) - 呼吸困难 (Hūxī kùnnán) (Mandarin)

- Definition: Difficulty breathing or breathlessness, often associated with coughing, which can indicate respiratory or cardiovascular issues such as asthma, pneumonia, or heart failure.

23. Painful breathing (English) - Douleur à la respiration (French) - Dolor al respirar (Spanish) - Schmerzen beim Atmen (German) - Боль при дыхании (Russian) - 呼吸时疼痛 (Hūxī shí téngtòng) (Mandarin)

- Definition: Discomfort or pain experienced during inhalation or exhalation, often exacerbated by coughing, indicating conditions such as pleurisy, pneumonia, or pulmonary embolism.

24. Burning sensation in the chest (English) - Sensation de brûlure dans la poitrine (French) - Sensación de ardor en el pecho (Spanish) - Brennendes Gefühl in der Brust (German) - Жжение в груди (Russian) - 胸部灼热感 (Xiōngbù zhuórè gǎn) (Mandarin)

- Definition: Feeling of heat or discomfort in the chest, often associated with coughing and indicative of conditions such as acid reflux, esophagitis, or angina.

25. Sudden onset of cough (English) - Apparition soudaine de la toux (French) - Comienzo repentino de la tos (Spanish) - Plötzliches Auftreten von Husten (German) - Внезапное появление кашля (Russian) - 咳嗽突然发作 (Késou túrán fāzuò) (Mandarin)

   - Definition: Abrupt or unexpected start of coughing, often indicative of acute respiratory infections such as cold, flu, or bronchitis.

26. Coughing up blood (English) - Cracher du sang (French) - Tos con sangre (Spanish) - Blut husten (German) - Кашель с кровью (Russian) - 咳血 (Kéxiě) (Mandarin)

   - Definition: Expelling blood from the respiratory tract during coughing, which can indicate serious conditions such as lung cancer, tuberculosis, or pulmonary embolism.

27. Difficulty sleeping due to cough (English) - Difficulté à dormir à cause de la toux (French) - Dificultad para dormir debido a la tos (Spanish) - Schlafstörungen durch Husten (German) - Затруднение сна из-за кашля (Russian) - 咳嗽导致睡眠困难 (Késou dǎozhì shuìmián kùnnán) (Mandarin)

   - Definition: Trouble falling asleep or staying asleep due to persistent coughing, which can significantly impact sleep quality and overall well-being.

28. Coughing worse at night (English) - Toux pire la nuit (French) - Tos empeora por la noche (Spanish) - Nachts schlimmerer Husten (German) - Кашель усиливается ночью (Russian) - 咳嗽夜间加重 (Késou yèjiān jiāzhòng) (Mandarin)

   - Definition: Cough that becomes more severe or frequent during the nighttime hours, often disrupting sleep and indicating conditions such as asthma, postnasal drip, or gastroesophageal reflux disease (GERD).

29. Fatigue with cough (English) - Fatigue avec toux (French) - Fatiga con tos (Spanish) - Müdigkeit mit Husten (German) - Усталость с кашлем (Russian) - 咳嗽疲劳 (Késou píláo) (Mandarin)

- Definition: Feeling of tiredness or exhaustion accompanied by coughing, which can be a symptom of an underlying infection or chronic respiratory condition.

30. Coughing up green or yellow mucus (English) - Cracher des glaires vertes ou jaunes (French) - Tos con mucosidad verde o amarilla (Spanish) - Grünen oder gelben Schleim husten (German) - Кашель с выделением зеленой или желтой мокроты (Russian) - 咳出绿色或黄色痰 (Ké chū lǜsè huò huángsè tán) (Mandarin)

- Definition: Expelling green or yellow-colored mucus or phlegm during coughing, which can indicate a bacterial infection such as bronchitis or pneumonia.

31. Coughing with a metallic taste (English) - Toux avec un goût métallique (French) - Tos con sabor metálico (Spanish) - Husten mit metallischem Geschmack (German) - Кашель с металлическим привкусом (Russian) - 咳嗽带有金属味 (Késou dàiyǒu jīnshǔ wèi) (Mandarin)

- Definition: Experiencing a metallic taste in the mouth during coughing, often indicating the presence of blood or bleeding in the respiratory tract.

32. Deep cough (English) - Toux profonde (French) - Tos profunda (Spanish) - Tiefer Husten (German) - Глубокий кашель (Russian) - 深咳 (Shēn késou) (Mandarin)

- Definition: Cough characterized by a low-pitched, resonant sound and originating from the lower respiratory tract, often indicative of conditions such as bronchitis, pneumonia, or lung disease.

33. Rhythmic cough (English) - Toux rythmique (French) - Tos rítmica (Spanish) - Rhythmischer Husten (German) - Ритмичный кашель (Russian) - 有规律的咳嗽 (Yǒu guīlǜ de késou) (Mandarin)

- Definition: Cough with a regular, repetitive pattern or cadence, often associated with conditions such as pertussis (whooping cough) or chronic bronchitis.

34. Breathlessness during coughing (English) - Essoufflement pendant la toux (French) - Falta de aire al toser (Spanish) - Atemnot beim Husten (German) - Одышка во время кашля (Russian) - 咳嗽时气短 (Késou shí qìduǎn) (Mandarin)

   - Definition: Feeling of shortness of breath or difficulty breathing that occurs concurrently with coughing, indicating respiratory distress or airway obstruction.

35. Dry, hacking cough (English) - Toux sèche et rauque (French) - Tos seca y persistente (Spanish) - Trockener, rauer Husten (German) - Сухой, хриплый кашель (Russian) - 干咳，剧咳 (Gān késou, jù késou) (Mandarin)

   - Definition: Persistent, harsh cough without production of mucus or phlegm, often caused by irritation or inflammation in the throat or airways.

36. Excessive coughing (English) - Toux excessive (French) - Tos excesiva (Spanish) - Übermäßiges Husten (German) - Чрезмерный кашель (Russian) - 过度咳嗽 (Guòdù késou) (Mandarin)

   - Definition: Abnormally frequent or prolonged coughing episodes, often indicative of underlying respiratory infections, allergies, or chronic conditions.

37. Difficulty speaking due to cough (English) - Difficulté à parler à cause de la toux (French) - Dificultad para hablar debido a la tos (Spanish) - Schwierigkeiten beim Sprechen aufgrund von Husten (German) - Затруднения при разговоре из-за кашля (Russian) - 由于咳嗽而说话困难 (Yóu yú késou ér shuōhuà kùnnán) (Mandarin)

   - Definition: Trouble articulating words or speaking clearly due to persistent coughing, which can affect communication and indicate significant throat or respiratory irritation.

38. Chronic cough (English) - Toux chronique (French) - Tos crónica (Spanish) - Chronischer Husten (German) - Хронический кашель (Russian) - 慢性咳嗽 (Màn xìng késou) (Mandarin)

- Definition: Persistent cough lasting for more than eight weeks, often indicating an underlying medical condition such as asthma, chronic bronchitis, or gastroesophageal reflux disease (GERD).

39. Difficulty concentrating due to cough (English) - Difficulté à se concentrer à cause de la toux (French) - Dificultad para concentrarse debido a la tos (Spanish) - Konzentrationsschwierigkeiten aufgrund von Husten (German) - Затруднения сосредоточиться из-за кашля (Russian) - 由于咳嗽而注意力难以集中 (Yóu yú késou ér zhùyìlì nányǐ jízhōng) (Mandarin)

- Definition: Inability to focus or maintain attention due to frequent coughing, which can disrupt daily activities and productivity.

40. Throat irritation with cough (English) - Irritation de la gorge avec toux (French) - Irritación de la garganta con tos (Spanish) - Reizung des Halses beim Husten (German) - Раздражение горла при кашле (Russian) - 咳嗽引起的喉咙不适 (Késou yǐnqǐ de hóulóng bùshì) (Mandarin)

- Definition: Sensation of scratchiness, dryness, or discomfort in the throat, often exacerbated by coughing, which can result from respiratory infections, allergies, or environmental irritants.

41. Coughing up foam (English) - Cracher de la mousse (French) - Tos con espuma (Spanish) - Schaum husten (German) - Кашель с пеной (Russian) - 咳白沫 (Ké bái mò) (Mandarin)

- Definition: Expelling frothy or bubbly substance during coughing, which can indicate conditions such as pulmonary edema, heart failure, or aspiration pneumonia.

42. Coughing fits triggered by laughter (English) - Accès de toux déclenchés par le rire (French) - Ataques de tos desencadenados por la risa (Spanish) - Hustenanfälle durch Lachen ausgelöst (German) - Приступы кашля, вызванные смехом (Russian) - 咳嗽发作由笑触发 (Késou fāzuò yóu xiào chùfā) (Mandarin)

- Definition: Episodes of intense coughing triggered by laughter or other emotional stimuli, often indicative of pertussis (whooping cough) or other respiratory conditions.

43. Coughing with a sore chest (English) - Toux avec une poitrine douloureuse (French) - Tos con dolor en el pecho (Spanish) - Husten mit schmerzender Brust (German) - Кашель с болезненной грудью (Russian) - 咳嗽伴胸痛 (Késou bàn xiōng tòng) (Mandarin)

- Definition: Cough accompanied by pain or discomfort in the chest area, which can indicate conditions such as pleurisy, costochondritis, or rib fracture.

44. Persistent tickle in the throat leading to cough (English) - Chatouillement persistant dans la gorge entraînant une toux (French) - Cosquilleo persistente en la garganta que provoca tos (Spanish) - Anhaltendes Kitzeln im Hals, das zu Husten führt (German) - Постоянное щекотание в горле, вызывающее кашель (Russian) - 持续的喉咙痒导致咳嗽 (Chíxù de hóulóng yǎng dǎozhì késou) (Mandarin)

- Definition: Continuous sensation of irritation or tickling in the throat, resulting in persistent coughing reflex, often seen in conditions such as postnasal drip or allergic rhinitis.

45. Coughing with chest heaviness (English) - Toux avec une sensation de lourdeur dans la poitrine (French) - Tos con sensación de opresión en el pecho (Spanish) - Husten mit Brustschwere (German) - Кашель с ощущением тяжести в груди (Russian) - 咳嗽伴胸闷 (Késou bàn xiōng mèn) (Mandarin)

- Definition: Cough accompanied by a feeling of pressure or heaviness in the chest, indicating possible bronchial constriction, asthma exacerbation, or cardiac issues.

46. Coughing fits after eating (English) - Accès de toux après avoir mangé (French) - Ataques de tos después de comer (Spanish) - Hustenanfälle nach dem Essen (German) - Приступы кашля после еды (Russian) - 饭后咳嗽 (Fàn hòu késou) (Mandarin)

- Definition: Episodes of intense coughing occurring shortly after meals, which can be indicative of gastroesophageal reflux disease (GERD), aspiration, or food allergies.

47. Wheezing during coughing (English) - Sifflement pendant la toux (French) - Sibilancias durante la tos (Spanish) - Pfeifen beim Husten (German) - Хрипы во время кашля (Russian) - 咳嗽时有喘鸣 (Késou shí yǒu chuǎnmíng) (Mandarin)

   - Definition: Production of high-pitched whistling sounds during coughing, often indicative of narrowed airways or bronchospasm associated with asthma or chronic obstructive pulmonary disease (COPD).

48. Coughing with a runny nose (English) - Toux avec un nez qui coule (French) - Tos con secreción nasal (Spanish) - Husten mit laufender Nase (German) - Кашель с насморком (Russian) - 咳嗽伴流鼻涕 (Késou bàn liú bítì) (Mandarin)

   - Definition: Cough accompanied by nasal discharge or a runny nose, often indicative of upper respiratory tract infections such as the common cold or sinus

49. Coughing with difficulty swallowing (English) - Toux avec difficulté à avaler (French) - Tos con dificultad para tragar (Spanish) - Husten mit Schluckbeschwerden (German) - Кашель с затруднением глотания (Russian) - 咳嗽伴有吞咽困难 (Késou bàn yǒu tūnyàn kùnnán) (Mandarin)

   - Definition: Experiencing pain or discomfort while swallowing accompanied by coughing, which can be indicative of conditions such as pharyngitis, tonsillitis, or esophagitis.

50. Coughing with a metallic smell (English) - Toux avec une odeur métallique (French) - Tos con olor metálico (Spanish) - Husten mit metallischem Geruch (German) - Кашель с металлическим запахом (Russian) - 咳嗽带金属气味 (Késou dài jīnshǔ qìwèi) (Mandarin)

   - Definition: Experiencing a metallic odor while coughing, often indicating the presence of blood in the respiratory tract or a metallic foreign body.

51. Coughing with chest congestion (English) - Toux avec congestion thoracique (French) - Tos con congestión torácica

(Spanish) - Husten mit Brustenge (German) - Кашель с загрудинной конгестией (Russian) - 咳嗽伴胸部充血 (Késou bàn xiōngbù chōngxiě) (Mandarin)

- Definition: Cough accompanied by a feeling of fullness or tightness in the chest due to the accumulation of mucus or fluid in the lungs.

52. Coughing with headache (English) - Toux avec mal de tête (French) - Tos con dolor de cabeza (Spanish) - Husten mit Kopfschmerzen (German) - Кашель с головной болью (Russian) - 咳嗽伴头痛 (Késou bàn tóutòng) (Mandarin)

- Definition: Experiencing head pain or discomfort concurrent with coughing, which can be indicative of conditions such as sinusitis, tension headache, or intracranial pressure.

53. Coughing with fever (English) - Toux avec fièvre (French) - Tos con fiebre (Spanish) - Husten mit Fieber (German) - Кашель с лихорадкой (Russian) - 咳嗽伴发烧 (Késou bàn fāshāo) (Mandarin)

- Definition: Presence of elevated body temperature or fever concurrent with coughing, which can indicate underlying infections such as influenza, pneumonia, or bronchitis.

54. Coughing with chills (English) - Toux avec frissons (French) - Tos con escalofríos (Spanish) - Husten mit Schüttelfrost (German) - Кашель с ознобом (Russian) - 咳嗽伴发冷 (Késou bàn fālěng) (Mandarin)

- Definition: Experiencing episodes of shivering or feeling cold accompanied by coughing, which can be indicative of systemic infections or fever.

55. Coughing with body aches (English) - Toux avec courbatures (French) - Tos con dolores corporales (Spanish) - Husten mit Körperschmerzen (German) - Кашель с болями в теле (Russian) - 咳嗽伴全身酸痛 (Késou bàn quánshēn suāntòng) (Mandarin)

- Definition: Experiencing generalized muscle pain or body aches concurrent with coughing, often indicative of systemic infections such as influenza or respiratory syncytial virus (RSV).

56. Coughing with shortness of breath (English) - Toux avec essoufflement (French) - Tos con falta de aire (Spanish) - Husten mit Atemnot (German) - Кашель с одышкой (Russian) - 咳嗽伴气短 (Késou bàn qìduǎn) (Mandarin)

- Definition: Experiencing breathlessness or difficulty breathing concurrent with coughing, which can indicate underlying respiratory or cardiac issues such as asthma, pneumonia, or heart failure.

57. Coughing with nasal congestion (English) - Toux avec congestion nasale (French) - Tos con congestión nasal (Spanish) - Husten mit Nasenverstopfung (German) - Кашель с насальной заложенность

8. HOSPITAL ROOM FURNITURE IN THE HOSPITAL

SOME GENERAL TERMS

1. Doctor - Médecin (French), Médico (Spanish), Arzt (German), Врач (Russian), 医生 (Mandarin)

2. Nurse - Infirmière (French), Enfermera (Spanish), Krankenschwester (German), медсестра (Russian), 护士 (Mandarin)

3. Patient - Patient (French), Paciente (Spanish), Patient (German), пациент (Russian), 病人 (Mandarin)

4. Hospital - Hôpital (French), Hospital (Spanish), Krankenhaus (German), больница (Russian), 医院 (Mandarin)

5. Surgery - Chirurgie (French), Cirugía (Spanish), Chirurgie (German), хирургия (Russian), 手術 (Mandarin)

6. Medicine - Médicament (French), Medicina (Spanish), Medikament (German), лекарство (Russian), 药物 (Mandarin)

7. Prescription - Ordonnance (French), Receta médica (Spanish), Rezept (German), рецепт (Russian), 处方 (Mandarin)

8. Symptom - Symptôme (French), Síntoma (Spanish), Symptom (German), симптом (Russian), 症状 (Mandarin)

9. Diagnosis - Diagnostic (French), Diagnóstico (Spanish), Diagnose (German), диагноз (Russian), 诊断 (Mandarin)

10. Treatment - Traitement (French), Tratamiento (Spanish), Behandlung (German), лечение (Russian), 治疗 (Mandarin)

11. Prevention - Prévention (French), Prevención (Spanish), Vorbeugung (German), профилактика (Russian), 预防 (Mandarin)

12. Vaccine - Vaccin (French), Vacuna (Spanish), Impfstoff (German), вакцина (Russian), 疫苗 (Mandarin)

13. Infection - Infection (French), Infección (Spanish), Infektion (German), инфекция (Russian), 感染 (Mandarin)

14. Fever - Fièvre (French), Fiebre (Spanish), Fieber (German), лихорадочность (Russian), 发烧 (Mandarin)

15. Pain - Douleur (French), Dolor (Spanish), Schmerz (German), болезненность (Russian), 疼痛 (Mandarin)

16. Allergy - Allergie (French), Alergia (Spanish), Allergie (German), аллергия (Russian), 过敏 (Mandarin)

17. Antibiotics - Antibiotiques (French), Antibióticos (Spanish), Antibakterielle Mittel (German), антибиотики (Russian), 抗生素 (Mandarin)

18. Lab test - Tests de laboratoire (French), Análisis de laboratorio (Spanish), Laboratorietests (German), лабораторные тесты (Russian), 实验室测试 (Mandarin)

19. Imaging - Imagerie (French), Imagenología (Spanish), Bildgebung (German), изобразительная диагностика (Russian), 图像学 (Mandarin)

20. Emergency - Urgence (French), Emergencia (Spanish), Notfall (German), чрезвычайная ситуация (Russian), 紧急情况 (Mandarin)

1. Fever

   - French: Fièvre

   - Spanish: Fiebre

   - German: Fieber

   - Russian: Жар (Zhar)

   - Mandarin: 发烧 (fāshāo)

   - Definition: Abnormal elevation of body temperature, often a sign of illness.

2. Pain

   - French: Douleur

   - Spanish: Dolor

   - German: Schmerz

   - Russian: Боль (Bol')

   - Mandarin: 疼痛 (téngtòng)

   - Definition: Unpleasant physical sensation caused by injury or illness.

3. Cough

   - French: Toux

   - Spanish: Tos

   - German: Husten

   - Russian: Кашель (Kashel')

   - Mandarin: 咳嗽 (késòu)

   - Definition: Expulsion of air from the lungs through the mouth due to irritation or infection.

4. Headache

   - French: Mal de tête

   - Spanish: Dolor de cabeza

   - German: Kopfschmerzen

   - Russian: Головная боль (Golovnaya bol')

   - Mandarin: 头痛 (tóutòng)

   - Definition: Pain or discomfort in the head or upper neck.

5. Nausea

   - French: Nausée

   - Spanish: Náuseas

   - German: Übelkeit

   - Russian: Тошнота (Toshnota)

   - Mandarin: 恶心 (ěxīn)

   - Definition: Feeling of discomfort or queasiness in the stomach, often preceding vomiting.

6. Diarrhea

   - French: Diarrhée

   - Spanish: Diarrea

   - German: Durchfall

   - Russian: Понос (Ponos)

   - Mandarin: 腹泻 (fùxiè)

   - Definition: Frequent and watery bowel movements.

7. Vomiting

- French: Vomissement

  - Spanish: Vómito

  - German: Erbrechen

  - Russian: Рвота (Rvota)

  - Mandarin: 呕吐 (ǒutù)

  - Definition: Forceful expulsion of stomach contents through the mouth.

8. Shortness of breath

  - French: Essoufflement

  - Spanish: Falta de aire

  - German: Atemnot

  - Russian: Одышка (Odyshka)

  - Mandarin: 呼吸困难 (hūxī kùnnán)

  - Definition: Difficulty breathing or a sensation of not getting enough air.

9. Fatigue

  - French: Fatigue

  - Spanish: Fatiga

  - German: Müdigkeit

  - Russian: Усталость (Ustalost')

  - Mandarin: 疲劳 (píláo)

  - Definition: Extreme tiredness or exhaustion.

10. Rash

  - French: Éruption cutanée

- Spanish: Erupción cutánea

- German: Hautausschlag

- Russian: Сыпь (Syp')

- Mandarin: 皮疹 (pízhěn)

- Definition: Change in the skin's appearance, often characterized by redness, bumps, or itching.

11. Swelling

- French: Gonflement

- Spanish: Hinchazón

- German: Schwellung

- Russian: Отек (Otek)

- Mandarin: 肿胀 (zhǒngzhàng)

- Definition: Enlargement or puffiness of a body part due to fluid accumulation.

12. Bruise

- French: Bleu

- Spanish: Moretón

- German: Bluterguss

- Russian: Синяк (Sinyak)

- Mandarin: 擦伤 (cāshāng)

- Definition: Discoloration of the skin caused by bleeding underneath due to trauma.

13. Infection

- French: Infection

- Spanish: Infección

  - German: Infektion

  - Russian: Инфекция (Infektsiya)

  - Mandarin: 感染 (gǎnrǎn)

  - Definition: Invasion and multiplication of microorganisms in body tissues, causing harm.

14. Allergy

  - French: Allergie

  - Spanish: Alergia

  - German: Allergie

  - Russian: Аллергия (Allergiya)

  - Mandarin: 过敏 (guòmǐn)

  - Definition: Hypersensitivity reaction to a foreign substance, triggering an immune response.

15. Sore throat

  - French: Mal de gorge

  - Spanish: Dolor de garganta

  - German: Halsschmerzen

  - Russian: Боль в горле (Bol' v gorle)

  - Mandarin: 喉咙痛 (hóulóng tòng)

  - Definition: Pain or irritation in the throat, often worsened by swallowing.

16. Heartburn

  - French: Brûlures d'estomac

- Spanish: Acidez estomacal

- German: Sodbrennen

- Russian: изжога (Izzhoga)

- Mandarin: 烧心 (shāo xīn)

- Definition: Burning sensation in the chest, caused by stomach acid refluxing into the esophagus.

17. Fainting

- French: Évanouissement

- Spanish: Desmayo

- German: Ohnmacht

- Russian: Обморок (Obmorok)

- Mandarin: 昏倒 (hūndǎo)

- Definition: Temporary loss of consciousness due to insufficient blood flow to the brain.

18. Stomach ache

- French: Mal de ventre

- Spanish: Dolor de estómago

- German: Bauchschmerzen

- Russian: Боль в животе (Bol' v zhivote)

- Mandarin: 胃痛 (wèitòng)

- Definition: Pain or discomfort in the abdomen.

19. Constipation

- French: Constipation

- Spanish: Estreñimiento

- German: Verstopfung

- Russian: Запор (Zapor)

- Mandarin: 便秘 (biànmì)

- Definition: Difficulty or infrequent bowel movements, often associated with hard stools.

20. Dizziness

- French: Vertige

- Spanish: Mareo

- German: Schwindel

21. High blood pressure

- French: Hypertension artérielle

- Spanish: Presión arterial alta

- German: Bluthochdruck

- Russian: Высокое давление (Vysokoye davleniye)

- Mandarin: 高血压 (gāo xuèyā)

- Definition: Elevated force of blood against the walls of arteries, increasing the risk of heart disease and stroke.

22. Low blood pressure

- French: Hypotension artérielle

- Spanish: Presión arterial baja

- German: Niedriger Blutdruck

- Russian: Низкое давление (Nizkoye davleniye)

   - Mandarin: 低血压 (dī xuèyā)

   - Definition: Abnormally low force of blood against the walls of arteries, leading to dizziness and fainting.

23. Urinary tract infection (UTI)

   - French: Infection urinaire

   - Spanish: Infección del tracto urinario

   - German: Harnwegsinfektion

   - Russian: Инфекция мочевого пузыря (Infektsiya mochevogo puzyrya)

   - Mandarin: 尿路感染 (niàolù gǎnrǎn)

   - Definition: Infection affecting any part of the urinary system, including the kidneys, bladder, ureters, and urethra.

24. Kidney stones

   - French: Calculs rénaux

   - Spanish: Cálculos renales

   - German: Nierensteine

   - Russian: Мочекаменная болезнь (Mochekamennaya bolezn')

   - Mandarin: 肾结石 (shèn jiéshí)

   - Definition: Hard deposits of minerals and salts that form in the kidneys and can cause severe pain when passing through the urinary tract.

25. Diabetes

   - French: Diabète

   - Spanish: Diabetes

- German: Diabetes

- Russian: Диабет (Diabet)

- Mandarin: 糖尿病 (táng niàobìng)

- Definition: Chronic condition characterized by high levels of sugar (glucose) in the blood, resulting from inadequate insulin production or ineffective use of insulin by the body.

26. Stroke

- French: Accident vasculaire cérébral (AVC)

- Spanish: Accidente cerebrovascular (ACV)

- German: Schlaganfall

- Russian: Инсульт (Insult)

- Mandarin: 中风 (zhōngfēng)

- Definition: Sudden interruption of blood supply to the brain, leading to brain damage and potentially permanent neurological deficits.

27. Heart attack

- French: Crise cardiaque

- Spanish: Ataque al corazón

- German: Herzinfarkt

- Russian: Инфаркт миокарда (Infarkt miokarda)

- Mandarin: 心脏病发作 (xīnzàng bìng fāzuò)

- Definition: Sudden blockage of blood flow to the heart, resulting in damage to heart muscle tissue.

28. Asthma

- French: Asthme

- Spanish: Asma

- German: Asthma

- Russian: Астма (Astma)

- Mandarin: 哮喘 (xiāochuǎn)

- Definition: Chronic respiratory condition characterized by inflammation and narrowing of the airways, leading to wheezing, coughing, and difficulty breathing.

29. Arthritis

- French: Arthrite

- Spanish: Artritis

- German: Arthritis

- Russian: Артрит (Artrit)

- Mandarin: 关节炎 (guānjié yán)

- Definition: Inflammation of one or more joints, causing pain, swelling, and stiffness.

30. Cancer

- French: Cancer

- Spanish: Cáncer

- German: Krebs

- Russian: Рак (Rak)

- Mandarin: 癌症 (áizhèng)

- Definition: Disease characterized by the uncontrolled growth and spread of abnormal cells, potentially invading other tissues and organs.

31. Anemia

- French: Anémie

- Spanish: Anemia

- German: Anämie

- Russian: Анемия (Anemiya)

- Mandarin: 贫血 (pínxiě)

- Definition: Condition characterized by a deficiency of red blood cells or hemoglobin in the blood, leading to fatigue and weakness.

32. Hypothyroidism

- French: Hypothyroïdie

- Spanish: Hipotiroidismo

- German: Hypothyreose

- Russian: Гипотиреоз (Gipotireoz)

- Mandarin: 甲状腺功能减退 (jiǎzhuàngxiàn gōngnéng jiǎntuì)

- Definition: Condition where the thyroid gland does not produce enough thyroid hormone, resulting in fatigue, weight gain, and other symptoms.

33. Hyperthyroidism

- French: Hyperthyroïdie

- Spanish: Hipertiroidismo

- German: Hyperthyreose

- Russian: Гипертиреоз (Giperpireoz)

- Mandarin: 甲状腺功能亢进 (jiǎzhuàngxiàn gōngnéng kàngjìn)

- Definition: Condition where the thyroid gland produces an excess of thyroid hormone, leading to weight loss, rapid heartbeat, and other symptoms.

34. Concussion

- French: Commotion cérébrale

- Spanish: Conmoción cerebral

- German: Gehirnerschütterung

- Russian: Сотрясение мозга (Sotryaseniye mozga)

- Mandarin: 脑震荡 (nǎo zhèn dàng)

- Definition: Mild traumatic brain injury caused by a blow to the head, resulting in temporary loss of normal brain function.

35. Gastroenteritis

- French: Gastro-entérite

- Spanish: Gastroenteritis

- German: Gastroenteritis

- Russian: Гастроэнтерит (Gastroenterit)

- Mandarin: 肠胃炎 (chángwèiyán)

- Definition: Inflammation of the stomach and intestines, typically causing diarrhea, vomiting, and abdominal pain.

36. Pneumonia

- French: Pneumonie

- Spanish: Neumonía

- German: Lungenentzündung

- Russian: Пневмония (Pnevmoniya)

- Mandarin: 肺炎 (fèiyán)

- Definition: Infection that inflames air sacs in one or both lungs, causing cough, fever, and difficulty breathing.

37. Cholesterol

   - French: Cholestérol

   - Spanish: Colesterol

   - German: Cholesterin

   - Russian: Холестерин (Kholesterin)

   - Mandarin: 胆固醇 (dǎngùchún)

   - Definition: Waxy substance found in blood, high levels of which can increase the risk of heart disease.

38. Obesity

   - French: Obésité

   - Spanish: Obesidad

   - German: Fettleibigkeit

   - Russian: Ожирение (Ozhireniye)

   - Mandarin: 肥胖 (féipàng)

   - Definition: Condition characterized by excess body fat accumulation, increasing the risk of various health problems.

39. Depression

   - French: Dépression

   - Spanish: Depresión

   - German: Depression

   - Russian: Депрессия (Depressiya)

   - Mandarin: 抑郁症 (yìyù zhèng)

   - Definition: Mood disorder causing persistent feelings of sadness, hopelessness, and loss of interest in activities.

40. Anxiety

   - French: Anxiété

   - Spanish: Ansiedad

   - German: Angst

   - Russian: Тревожность (Trevozhnost')

   - Mandarin: 焦虑 (jiāolǜ)

   - Definition: Persistent worry, fear, or apprehension about future events, often accompanied by physical symptoms such as palpitations or sweating.

41. Insomnia

   - French: Insomnie

   - Spanish: Insomnio

   - German: Schlaflosigkeit

   - Russian: Бессонница (Bessonnitsa)

   - Mandarin: 失眠 (shīmián)

   - Definition: Persistent difficulty falling asleep or staying asleep, leading to inadequate rest and daytime impairment.

42. Hypertension

   - French: Hypertension

   - Spanish: Hipertensión

   - German: Hypertonie

   - Russian: Гипертония (Gipertoniya)

- Mandarin: 高血压 (gāo xuèyā)

- Definition: Medical condition characterized by elevated blood pressure in the arteries, increasing the risk of cardiovascular diseases.

43. Hypotension

- French: Hypotension

- Spanish: Hipotensión

- German: Hypotonie

- Russian: Гипотония (Gipotoniya)

- Mandarin: 低血压 (dī xuèyā)

- Definition: Medical condition characterized by abnormally low blood pressure, often resulting in dizziness and fainting.

44. Jaundice

- French: Jaunisse

- Spanish: Ictericia

- German: Gelbsucht

- Russian: Желтуха (Zheltukha)

- Mandarin: 黄疸 (huángdǎn)

- Definition: Yellow discoloration of the skin and whites of the eyes, caused by excess bilirubin in the blood.

45. Seizure

- French: Crise convulsive

- Spanish: Convulsión

- German: Krampfanfall

- Russian: Припадок (Pripadok)

- Mandarin: 癫痫发作 (diānxián fāzuò)

- Definition: Sudden, uncontrolled electrical disturbance in the brain, resulting in abnormal behavior, movements, and sensations.

46. Migraine

- French: Migraine

- Spanish: Migraña

- German: Migräne

- Russian: Мигрень (Migren')

- Mandarin: 偏头痛 (piāntóutòng)

- Definition: Recurrent throbbing headache, often accompanied by nausea, vomiting, and sensitivity to light and sound.

47. Gastric ulcer

- French: Ulcère gastrique

- Spanish: Úlcera gástrica

- German: Magengeschwür

- Russian: Язва желудка (Yazva zheludka)

- Mandarin: 胃溃疡 (wèi kuìyáng)

- Definition: Open sore that forms on the lining of the stomach, causing abdominal pain and discomfort.

48. Cataract

- French: Cataracte

- Spanish: Catarata

- German: Grauer Star

- Russian: Катаракта (Katarakta)

- Mandarin: 白内障 (báinèizhàng)

   - Definition: Clouding of the eye's natural lens, leading to blurry vision and eventual vision loss if left untreated.

49. Gout

   - French: Goutte

   - Spanish: Gota

   - German: Gicht

   - Russian: Подагра (Podagra)

   - Mandarin: 痛风 (tòngfēng)

   - Definition: Form of arthritis characterized by sudden, severe attacks of pain, redness, and swelling in the joints, often affecting the big toe.

50. Osteoporosis

   - French: Ostéoporose

   - Spanish: Osteoporosis

   - German: Osteoporose

   - Russian: Остеопороз (Osteoporoz)

   - Mandarin: 骨质疏松症 (gǔzhì shūsōngzhèng)

   - Definition: Condition characterized by fragile and porous bones, increasing the risk of fractures.

51. Anorexia

   - French: Anorexie

   - Spanish: Anorexia

- German: Anorexie

- Russian: Анорексия (Anoreksiya)

- Mandarin: 厌食症 (yànshízhèng)

- Definition: Eating disorder characterized by an intense fear of gaining weight and a distorted body image, leading to self-imposed starvation and excessive weight loss.

52. Bulimia

- French: Boulimie

- Spanish: Bulimia

- German: Bulimie

- Russian: Булимия (Bulimiya)

- Mandarin: 暴食症 (bàoshízhèng)

- Definition: Eating disorder characterized by recurrent episodes of binge eating followed by purging behaviors such as vomiting, fasting, or excessive exercise.

53. Schizophrenia

- French: Schizophrénie

- Spanish: Esquizofrenia

- German: Schizophrenie

- Russian: Шизофрения (Shizofreniya)

- Mandarin: 精神分裂症 (jīngshén fēnlièzhèng)

- Definition: Chronic mental disorder characterized by distorted thinking, hallucinations, delusions, and impaired social functioning.

54. Panic attack

- French: Crise de panique

- Spanish: Ataque de pánico

- German: Panikattacke

- Russian: Паническая атака (Panicheskaya ataka)

- Mandarin: 恐慌发作 (kǒnghuāng fāzuò)

- Definition: Sudden onset of intense fear or discomfort, accompanied by physical symptoms such as rapid heartbeat, sweating, trembling, and shortness of breath.

55. Rheumatoid arthritis

- French: Polyarthrite rhumatoïde

- Spanish: Artritis reumatoide

- German: Rheumatoide Arthritis

- Russian: Ревматоидный артрит (Revmatoidnyy artrit)

- Mandarin: 类风湿性关节炎 (lèifēngshīxìng guānjiéyán)

- Definition: Chronic inflammatory disorder affecting multiple joints, causing pain, swelling, stiffness, and potential joint deformity.

56. Chronic obstructive pulmonary disease (COPD)

- French: Maladie pulmonaire obstructive chronique (MPOC)

- Spanish: Enfermedad pulmonar obstructiva crónica (EPOC)

- German: Chronisch obstruktive Lungenerkrankung (COPD)

- Russian: Хроническое обструктивное заболевание легких (Khronicheskoye obstruktivnoye zabolevaniye legkikh)

- Mandarin: 慢性阻塞性肺疾病 (màn xìng zǔ sè xìng fèi jí bìng)

- Definition: Progressive lung disease characterized by airflow limitation, usually caused by exposure to irritants such as cigarette smoke, leading to symptoms like coughing, wheezing, and shortness of breath.

57. Glaucoma

- French: Glaucome
- Spanish: Glaucoma
- German: Glaukom
- Russian: Глаукома (Glaukoma)
- Mandarin: 青光眼 (qīng guāng yǎn)
- Definition: Eye condition characterized by increased pressure within the eye, damaging the optic nerve and leading to vision loss if left untreated.

58. Emphysema

- French: Emphysème
- Spanish: Enfisema
- German: Emphysem
- Russian: Эмфизема (Emfizema)
- Mandarin: 肺气肿 (fèiqìzhǒng)
- Definition: Lung condition characterized by damaged air sacs in the lungs, leading to difficulty breathing and reduced oxygen intake.

59. Multiple sclerosis (MS)

- French: Sclérose en plaques
- Spanish: Esclerosis múltiple
- German: Multiple Sklerose (MS)
- Russian: Множественная склероз (Mnozhestvennaya skleroz)
- Mandarin: 多发性硬化症 (duō fā xìng yìng huà zhèng)
- Definition: Chronic autoimmune disease affecting the central nervous system, causing a wide range of symptoms including

fatigue, weakness, numbness, and impaired coordination.

60. Parkinson's disease

   - French: Maladie de Parkinson

   - Spanish: Enfermedad de Parkinson

   - German: Parkinson-Krankheit

   - Russian: Болезнь Паркинсона (Bolezn' Parkinsona)

   - Mandarin: 帕金森病 (pàjīnsēn bìng)

   - Definition: Progressive nervous system disorder affecting movement, characterized by tremors, stiffness, and impaired balance and coordination.

61. Osteoarthritis

   - French: Ostéoarthrite

   - Spanish: Osteoartritis

   - German: Osteoarthritis

   - Russian: Остеоартроз (Osteoartroz)

   - Mandarin: 骨关节炎 (gǔ guānjié yán)

   - Definition: Degenerative joint disease characterized by the breakdown of joint cartilage and underlying bone, leading to pain, stiffness, and reduced mobility.

62. Epilepsy

   - French: Épilepsie

   - Spanish: Epilepsia

   - German: Epilepsie

   - Russian: Эпилепсия (Epilepsiya)

   - Mandarin: 癫痫病 (diānxián bìng)

- Definition: Neurological disorder characterized by recurrent seizures, which are sudden, uncontrolled electrical disturbances in the brain.

63. Fibromyalgia

   - French: Fibromyalgie

   - Spanish: Fibromialgia

   - German: Fibromyalgie

   - Russian: Фибромиалгия (Fibromialgiya)

   - Mandarin: 纤维肌痛综合症 (xiānwéi jī tòng zònghé zhèng)

   - Definition: Chronic disorder characterized by widespread musculoskeletal pain, fatigue, and tenderness in localized areas called tender points.

64. Crohn's disease

   - French: Maladie de Crohn

   - Spanish: Enfermedad de Crohn

   - German: Morbus Crohn

   - Russian: Болезнь Крона (Bolezn' Krona)

   - Mandarin: 克罗恩病 (kèluó'ēn bìng)

   - Definition: Inflammatory bowel disease causing inflammation of the digestive tract, leading to abdominal pain, diarrhea, weight loss, and fatigue.

65. Ulcerative colitis

   - French: Rectocolite hémorragique

   - Spanish: Colitis ulcerosa

   - German: Colitis ulcerosa

   - Russian: Язвенный колит (Yazvennyy kolit)

- Mandarin: 溃疡性结肠炎 (kuìyáng xìng jiécháng yán)

- Definition: Chronic inflammatory bowel disease characterized by inflammation and ulcers in the lining of the colon and rectum, leading to abdominal pain, diarrhea, and rectal bleeding.

66. Endometriosis

- French: Endométriose

- Spanish: Endometriosis

- German: Endometriose

- Russian: Эндометриоз (Endometrioz)

- Mandarin: 子宫内膜异位症 (zǐgōng nèimó yìwèi zhèng)

- Definition: Disorder where tissue similar to the lining of the uterus grows outside the uterus, causing pelvic pain, irregular menstruation, and infertility.

67. Polycystic ovary syndrome (PCOS)

- French: Syndrome des ovaires polykystiques (SOPK)

- Spanish: Síndrome de ovario poliquístico (SOP)

- German: Polyzystisches Ovarialsyndrom (PCOS)

- Russian: Поликистоз яичников (Polikistoz yaichnikov)

- Mandarin: 多囊卵巢综合征 (duō náng luǎncháo zònghé zhèng)

- Definition: Hormonal disorder in women of reproductive age, characterized by cysts in the ovaries, irregular menstrual cycles, and symptoms such as acne and hirsutism.

68. Hemorrhoids

- French: Hémorroïdes

- Spanish: Hemorroides

- German: Hämorrhoiden

- Russian: Геморрой (Gemorroy)

- Mandarin: 痔疮 (zhìchuāng)

- Definition: Swollen and inflamed veins in the rectum and anus, causing pain, itching, and bleeding during bowel movements.

69. Sleep apnea

- French: Apnée du sommeil

- Spanish: Apnea del sueño

- German: Schlafapnoe

- Russian: Апноэ сна (Apnoe sna)

- Mandarin: 睡眠呼吸暂停症 (shuìmián hūxī zàntíng zhèng)

- Definition: Sleep disorder characterized by pauses in breathing or shallow breaths during sleep, leading to fragmented sleep and daytime sleepiness.

70. Psoriasis

- French: Psoriasis

- Spanish: Psoriasis

- German: Psoriasis

- Russian: Псориаз (Psoriaz)

- Mandarin: 银屑病 (yínxuè bìng)

- Definition: Chronic autoimmune condition characterized by patches of thick, red skin covered with silvery scales, often affecting the elbows, knees, scalp, and lower back.

71. Hypoglycemia

   - French: Hypoglycémie

   - Spanish: Hipoglucemia

   - German: Hypoglykämie

   - Russian: Гипогликемия (Gipoglikemiya)

   - Mandarin: 低血糖 (dī xiětáng)

   - Definition: Condition characterized by abnormally low levels of glucose (sugar) in the blood, leading to symptoms such as dizziness, sweating, and confusion.

72. Hyperglycemia

   - French: Hyperglycémie

   - Spanish: Hiperglucemia

   - German: Hyperglykämie

   - Russian: Гипергликемия (Giperglikemiya)

   - Mandarin: 高血糖 (gāo xiětáng)

   - Definition: Condition characterized by abnormally high levels of glucose (sugar) in the blood, often associated with diabetes mellitus.

73. Obstructive sleep apnea

   - French: Apnée obstructive du sommeil

   - Spanish: Apnea obstructiva del sueño

   - German: Obstruktive Schlafapnoe

   - Russian: Обструктивная апноэ сна (Obstruktivnaya apnoe sna)

   - Mandarin: 阻塞性睡眠呼吸暂停症 (zǔsèxìng shuìmián hūxī zàntíng zhèng)

   - Definition: Sleep disorder characterized by repetitive episodes of complete or partial upper airway obstruction during sleep, leading to breathing pauses and disruptions in sleep.

74. Pancreatitis

   - French: Pancréatite

   - Spanish: Pancreatitis

   - German: Pankreatitis

   - Russian: Панкреатит (Pankreatit)

   - Mandarin: 胰腺炎 (yíxiàn yán)

   - Definition: Inflammation of the pancreas, causing severe abdominal pain, nausea, vomiting, and potentially life-threatening complications.

75. Celiac disease

   - French: Maladie cœliaque

   - Spanish: Enfermedad celíaca

   - German: Zöliakie

   - Russian: Болезнь Келия (Bolezn' Keliya)

   - Mandarin: 乳糜泻 (rǔmíxiè)

   - Definition: Autoimmune disorder triggered by gluten consumption, causing damage to the lining of the small intestine and leading to symptoms such as diarrhea, abdominal pain, and malabsorption of nutrients.

76. Sickle cell disease

   - French: Drépanocytose

   - Spanish: Anemia falciforme

   - German: Sichelzellenanämie

   - Russian: Серповидно-клеточная анемия (Serpovidnokletochnaya anemiya)

- Mandarin: 镰状细胞病 (liánzhuàng xìbāo bìng)

- Definition: Inherited blood disorder characterized by abnormal hemoglobin molecules, causing red blood cells to become rigid and sickle-shaped, leading to episodes of pain, anemia, and organ damage.

77. Hepatitis

- French: Hépatite

- Spanish: Hepatitis

- German: Hepatitis

- Russian: Гепатит (Gepatit)

- Mandarin: 肝炎 (gānyán)

- Definition: Inflammation of the liver, often caused by viral infection, alcohol consumption, or autoimmune disorders, leading to symptoms such as jaundice, fatigue, and abdominal pain.

78. Osteoporosis

- French: Ostéoporose

- Spanish: Osteoporosis

- German: Osteoporose

- Russian: Остеопороз (Osteoporoz)

- Mandarin: 骨质疏松症 (gǔzhì shūsōngzhèng)

- Definition: Condition characterized by fragile and porous bones, increasing the risk of fractures.

79. Meningitis

- French: Méningite

- Spanish: Meningitis

- German: Meningitis

- Russian: Менингит (Meningit)

- Mandarin: 脑膜炎 (nǎomó yán)

- Definition: Inflammation of the membranes (meninges) surrounding the brain and spinal cord, typically caused by infection, leading to symptoms such as headache, fever, and stiffness of the neck.

80. Gastritis

- French: Gastrite

- Spanish: Gastritis

- German: Gastritis

- Russian: Гастрит (Gastrit)

- Mandarin: 胃炎 (wèiyán)

- Definition: Inflammation of the lining of the stomach, often caused by infection, excessive alcohol consumption, or certain medications, leading to symptoms such as abdominal pain, nausea, and vomiting.

81. Hypothyroidism

- French: Hypothyroïdie

- Spanish: Hipotiroidismo

- German: Hypothyreose

- Russian: Гипотиреоз (Gipotireoz)

- Mandarin: 甲状腺功能减退 (jiǎzhuàngxiàn gōngnéng jiǎntuì)

- Definition: A medical condition where the thyroid gland does not produce enough thyroid hormone, leading to symptoms such as fatigue, weight gain, and cold intolerance.

82. Hyperthyroidism

   - French: Hyperthyroïdie

   - Spanish: Hipertiroidismo

   - German: Hyperthyreose

   - Russian: Гипертиреоз (Giperpireoz)

   - Mandarin: 甲状腺功能亢进 (jiǎzhuàngxiàn gōngnéng kàngjìn)

   - Definition: A medical condition where the thyroid gland produces an excess of thyroid hormone, leading to symptoms such as weight loss, rapid heartbeat, and heat intolerance.

83. Hernia

   - French: Hernie

   - Spanish: Hernia

   - German: Hernie

   - Russian: Грыжа (Gryzha)

   - Mandarin: 疝气 (shànqì)

   - Definition: A protrusion of an organ or tissue through an abnormal opening in the body wall, often causing a visible lump or bulge and sometimes pain or discomfort.

84. Ovarian cyst

   - French: Kyste ovarien

   - Spanish: Quiste ovárico

   - German: Ovarialzyste

   - Russian: Киста яичника (Kista yaitchnika)

- Mandarin: 卵巢囊肿 (luǎncháo nángzhǒng)

- Definition: A fluid-filled sac that forms on or inside the ovary, often causing abdominal pain, bloating, or changes in menstrual cycle.

85. Gallstones

   - French: Calculs biliaires

   - Spanish: Cálculos biliares

   - German: Gallensteine

   - Russian: Желчные камни (Zheltchnyye kamni)

   - Mandarin: 胆结石 (dǎn jiéshí)

- Definition: Hard deposits formed in the gallbladder or bile ducts, typically composed of cholesterol or bilirubin, causing severe abdominal pain, nausea, and vomiting.

86. Glomerulonephritis

   - French: Glomérulonéphrite

   - Spanish: Glomerulonefritis

   - German: Glomerulonephritis

   - Russian: Гломерулонефрит (Glomerulonefrit)

   - Mandarin: 肾小球肾炎 (shèn xiǎoqiú shènyán)

- Definition: Inflammation of the glomeruli in the kidneys, leading to proteinuria, hematuria, and impaired kidney function.

87. Diverticulitis

   - French: Diverticulite

   - Spanish: Diverticulitis

   - German: Divertikulitis

- Russian: Дивертикулит (Divertikulit)

- Mandarin: 憩室炎 (qìshì yán)

- Definition: Inflammation or infection of the diverticula, small pouches that can form in the lining of the digestive system, causing abdominal pain, fever, and changes in bowel habits.

88. Cirrhosis

- French: Cirrhose

- Spanish: Cirrosis

- German: Zirrhose

- Russian: Цирроз (Tsirroz)

- Mandarin: 肝硬化 (gān yìnghuà)

- Definition: Chronic liver disease characterized by the progressive scarring of liver tissue, leading to impaired liver function, jaundice, and complications such as ascites and hepatic encephalopathy.

89. Anemia

- French: Anémie

- Spanish: Anemia

- German: Anämie

- Russian: Анемия (Anemiya)

- Mandarin: 贫血 (pínxiě)

- Definition: A condition characterized by a deficiency of red blood cells or hemoglobin in the blood, leading to fatigue, weakness, and shortness of breath.

90. Appendicitis

- French: Appendicite

- Spanish: Apendicitis

- German: Appendizitis

- Russian: Аппендицит (Appenditsit)

- Mandarin: 阑尾炎 (lánwěi yán)

- Definition: Inflammation of the appendix, a small pouch attached to the large intestine, typically causing abdominal pain, nausea, vomiting, and fever.

91. Varicose veins

- French: Varices

- Spanish: Varices

- German: Krampfadern

- Russian: Варикозное расширение вен (Varikoznoye rasshireniye ven)

- Mandarin: 静脉曲张 (jìngmài qūzhāng)

- Definition: Enlarged and twisted veins, usually appearing in the legs, that can cause pain, swelling, and aching discomfort.

92. Gastroesophageal reflux disease (GERD)

- French: Reflux gastro-œsophagien (RGO)

- Spanish: Enfermedad por reflujo gastroesofágico (ERGE)

- German: Gastroösophagealer Reflux (GERD)

- Russian: Гастроэзофагеальный рефлюкс (GERD) (Gastroezofageal'nyy reflyuks)

- Mandarin: 胃食管反流病 (wèi shíguǎn fǎnliú bìng)

- Definition: A chronic digestive disorder where stomach acid flows back into the esophagus, causing heartburn, chest pain, and discomfort.

93. Benign prostatic hyperplasia (BPH)

   - French: Hyperplasie bénigne de la prostate (HBP)

   - Spanish: Hiperplasia benigna de próstata (HBP)

   - German: Benigne Prostatahyperplasie (BPH)

   - Russian: Доброкачественная гиперплазия простаты (Dobrokachestvennaya giperplaziya prostaty)

   - Mandarin: 良性前列腺增生 (liángxìng qiánlièxiàn zēngshēng)

   - Definition: Non-cancerous enlargement of the prostate gland, which can cause urinary symptoms such as frequent urination, urgency, and weak urine flow.

94. Systemic lupus erythematosus (SLE)

   - French: Lupus érythémateux disséminé (LED)

   - Spanish: Lupus eritematoso sistémico (LES)

   - German: Systemischer Lupus erythematodes (SLE)

   - Russian: Системная красная волчанка (Sistemnaya krasnaya volchanka)

   - Mandarin: 系统性红斑狼疮 (xìtǒngxìng hóngbān lángchuáng)

   - Definition: Autoimmune disease where the immune system attacks healthy tissues, leading to inflammation and damage to various organs and systems, including joints, skin, kidneys, and heart.

95. Hypertensive heart disease

   - French: Cardiopathie hypertensive

   - Spanish: Cardiopatía hipertensiva

- German: Hypertensive Herzerkrankung

- Russian: Гипертоническая болезнь сердца (Gipertonicheskaya bolezn' serdtsa)

- Mandarin: 高血压性心脏病 (gāo xuèyā xìng xīnzàng bìng)

- Definition: Heart conditions caused by long-term high blood pressure, which can lead to coronary artery disease, heart failure, and other complications.

96. Interstitial cystitis

- French: Cystite interstitielle

- Spanish: Cistitis intersticial

- German: Interstitielle Zystitis

- Russian: Интерстициальный цистит (Interstitsial'nyy tsistit)

- Mandarin: 间质性膀胱炎 (jiànzhìxìng pángguāng yán)

- Definition: Chronic bladder condition characterized by pelvic pain, urinary urgency, and frequency, often without bacterial infection.

97. Chronic kidney disease (CKD)

- French: Maladie rénale chronique (MRC)

- Spanish: Enfermedad renal crónica (ERC)

- German: Chronische Nierenkrankheit (CKD)

- Russian: Хроническая болезнь почек (Khronicheskaya bolezn' pochek)

- Mandarin: 慢性肾脏病 (màn xìng shènzàng bìng)

- Definition: Progressive loss of kidney function over time, leading to complications such as fluid retention, electrolyte imbalances, and anemia.

98. Chronic obstructive pulmonary disease (COPD)

   - French: Maladie pulmonaire obstructive chronique (MPOC)

   - Spanish: Enfermedad pulmonar obstructiva crónica (EPOC)

   - German: Chronisch obstruktive Lungenerkrankung (COPD)

   - Russian: Хроническое обструктивное заболевание легких (ХОЗЛ) (Khronicheskoye obstruktivnoye zabolevaniye legkikh)

   - Mandarin: 慢性阻塞性肺疾病 (màn xìng zǔ sè xìng fèi jí bìng)

   - Definition: Progressive lung disease characterized by airflow limitation, usually caused by exposure to irritants such as cigarette smoke, leading to symptoms like coughing, wheezing, and shortness of breath.

99. Diabetic neuropathy

   - French: Neuropathie diabétique

   - Spanish: Neuropatía diabética

   - German: Diabetische Neuropathie

   - Russian: Диабетическая нейропатия (Diabeticheskaya neyropatiya)

   - Mandarin: 糖尿病性神经病变 (tángniàobìngxìng shénjīng bìngbiàn)

   - Definition: Nerve damage caused by diabetes, leading to symptoms such as numbness, tingling, and pain in the affected areas, often in the hands and feet.

100. Dementia

   - French: Démence

   - Spanish: Demencia

   - German: Demenz

- Russian: Деменция (Dementsiya)

- Mandarin: 痴呆症 (chīdāizhèng)

- Definition: Progressive decline in cognitive function, including memory loss, reasoning, and judgment, often associated with aging or neurodegenerative diseases such as Alzheimer's.

101. Asthma

- French: Asthme

- Spanish: Asma

- German: Asthma

- Russian: Астма (Astma)

- Mandarin: 哮喘 (xiàochuǎn)

- Definition: Chronic respiratory condition characterized by inflammation and narrowing of the airways, leading to recurrent episodes of wheezing, coughing, chest tightness, and shortness of breath.

102. Urinary tract infection (UTI)

- French: Infection urinaire

- Spanish: Infección del tracto urinario (ITU)

- German: Harnwegsinfektion (HWI)

- Russian: Инфекция мочевыводящих путей (Infektsiya mochevyyvodyashchikh putey)

- Mandarin: 尿路感染 (niàolù gǎnrǎn)

- Definition: Infection involving the kidneys, ureters, bladder, or urethra, typically caused by bacteria, leading to symptoms such as urinary urgency, frequency, burning sensation, and lower abdominal pain.

103. Hypertension

- French: Hypertension artérielle

- Spanish: Hipertensión arterial

- German: Hypertonie

- Russian: Гипертония (Gipertoniy)

- Mandarin: 高血压 (gāo xuèyā)

- Definition: High blood pressure persistently elevated over time, increasing the risk of heart disease, stroke, and other complications.

104. Pancreatic cancer

- French: Cancer du pancréas

- Spanish: Cáncer de páncreas

- German: Bauchspeicheldrüsenkrebs

- Russian: Рак поджелудочной железы (Rak podzheludochnoy zhelezy)

- Mandarin: 胰腺癌 (yíxiàn ái)

- Definition: Malignant tumor originating in the pancreas, often diagnosed at an advanced stage, leading to symptoms such as abdominal pain, weight loss, jaundice, and digestive problems.

105. Deep vein thrombosis (DVT)

- French: Thrombose veineuse profonde (TVP)

- Spanish: Trombosis venosa profunda (TVP)

- German: Tiefe Venenthrombose (TVT)

- Russian: Глубокая венозная тромбоз (Glyubokaya venoznaya tromboz)

- Mandarin: 深静脉血栓 (shēn jìngmài xuèsuān)

- Definition: Formation of a blood clot (thrombus) in a deep vein, usually in the legs, leading to symptoms such as pain, swelling, warmth, and redness.

106. Myocardial infarction (heart attack)

- French: Infarctus du myocarde

- Spanish: Infarto de miocardio

- German: Herzinfarkt

- Russian: Инфаркт миокарда (Infarkt miokarda)

- Mandarin: 心肌梗死 (xīnjī gěngsǐ)

- Definition: Blockage of blood flow to the heart muscle, resulting in tissue damage or death, often presenting with chest pain, shortness of breath, and sweating.

107. Ovarian cancer

- French: Cancer de l'ovaire

- Spanish: Cáncer de ovario

- German: Eierstockkrebs

- Russian: Рак яичников (Rak yaichnikov)

- Mandarin: 卵巢癌 (luǎncháo ái)

- Definition: Cancerous growth originating in the ovaries, often diagnosed at an advanced stage, leading to symptoms such as abdominal bloating, pelvic pain, and changes in bowel habits.

108. Carpal tunnel syndrome

- French: Syndrome du canal carpien

- Spanish: Síndrome del túnel carpiano

- German: Karpaltunnelsyndrom

- Russian: Синдром карпального канала (Sindrom karpal'nogo kanala)

- Mandarin: 腕管综合征 (wànguǎn zònghé zhèng)

- Definition: Compression of the median nerve in the wrist, causing symptoms such as pain, numbness, and tingling in the hand and fingers.

109. Gastric ulcer

- French: Ulcère gastrique

- Spanish: Úlcera gástrica

- German: Magengeschwür

- Russian: Желудочная язва (Zheludochnaya yazva)

- Mandarin: 胃溃疡 (wèi kuìyáng)

- Definition: A sore or lesion that develops on the lining of the stomach, often caused by infection with Helicobacter pylori bacteria or long-term use of nonsteroidal anti-inflammatory drugs (NSAIDs).

110. Pneumonia

- French: Pneumonie

- Spanish: Neumonía

- German: Lungenentzündung

- Russian: Пневмония (Pnevmoniya)

- Mandarin: 肺炎 (fèiyán)

- Definition: Inflammation of the air sacs in one or both lungs, usually caused by infection with bacteria, viruses, or fungi, leading to symptoms such as cough, fever, chest pain, and difficulty breathing.

111. Gout

- French: Goutte

- Spanish: Gota

- German: Gicht

- Russian: Подагра (Podagra)

- Mandarin: 痛风 (tòngfēng)

- Definition: A form of arthritis characterized by sudden, severe attacks of pain, redness, swelling, and tenderness in the joints, typically affecting the big toe.

112. Menopause

- French: Ménopause

- Spanish: Menopausia

- German: Menopause

- Russian: Менопауза (Menopauza)

- Mandarin: 绝经期 (juéjīng qī)

- Definition: The natural cessation of menstruation and reproductive function in women, typically occurring around the age of 45 to 55, accompanied by symptoms such as hot flashes, mood swings, and vaginal dryness.

113. Fibroid

- French: Fibrome

- Spanish: Fibroma

- German: Fibrom

- Russian: Фиброма (Fibroma)

- Mandarin: 子宫肌瘤 (zǐgōng jīliú)

- Definition: Benign growth or tumor composed of fibrous tissue and muscle cells, usually found in the uterus (uterine fibroids), leading to symptoms such as pelvic pain, heavy menstrual bleeding, and urinary frequency.

114. Ectopic pregnancy

   - French: Grossesse extra-utérine

   - Spanish: Embarazo ectópico

   - German: Eileiterschwangerschaft

   - Russian: Эктопическая беременность (Ektopicheskaya beremennost')

   - Mandarin: 异位妊娠 (yìwèi rènshēn)

   - Definition: A pregnancy where the fertilized egg implants and grows outside the uterus, usually in the fallopian tube, leading to symptoms such as abdominal pain, vaginal bleeding, and dizziness.

115. Celiac disease

   - French: Maladie cœliaque

   - Spanish: Enfermedad celíaca

   - German: Zöliakie

   - Russian: Болезнь Келия (Bolezn' Keliya)

   - Mandarin: 乳糜泻 (rǔmíxiè)

   - Definition: An autoimmune disorder triggered by gluten consumption, causing damage to the lining of the small intestine and leading to symptoms such as diarrhea, abdominal pain, and malabsorption of nutrients.

116. Rheumatoid arthritis

   - French: Polyarthrite rhumatoïde

   - Spanish: Artritis reumatoide

   - German: Rheumatoide Arthritis

   - Russian: Ревматоидный артрит (Revmatoidnyy artrit)

- Mandarin: 类风湿性关节炎 (lèifēngshīxìng guānjié yán)

- Definition: A chronic inflammatory disorder affecting the joints, causing pain, stiffness, swelling, and deformity, typically affecting multiple joints symmetrically.

117. Hypothyroidism

- French: Hypothyroïdie

- Spanish: Hipotiroidismo

- German: Hypothyreose

- Russian: Гипотиреоз (Gipotireoz)

- Mandarin: 甲状腺功能减退 (jiǎzhuàngxiàn gōngnéng jiǎntuì)

- Definition: A medical condition where the thyroid gland does not produce enough thyroid hormone, leading to symptoms such as fatigue, weight gain, and cold intolerance.

118. Hyperthyroidism

- French: Hyperthyroïdie

- Spanish: Hipertiroidismo

- German: Hyperthyreose

- Russian: Гипертиреоз (Giperpireoz)

- Mandarin: 甲状腺功能亢进 (jiǎzhuàngxiàn gōngnéng kàngjìn)

- Definition: A medical condition where the thyroid gland produces an excess of thyroid hormone, leading to symptoms such as weight loss, rapid heartbeat, and heat intolerance.

119. Hernia

- French: Hernie

- Spanish: Hernia

- German: Hernie

- Russian: Грыжа (Gryzha)

- Mandarin: 疝气 (shànqì)

- Definition: A protrusion of an organ or tissue through an abnormal opening in the body wall, often causing a visible lump or bulge and sometimes pain or discomfort.

120. Ovarian cyst

- French: Kyste ovarien

- Spanish: Quiste ovárico

- German: Ovarialzyste

- Russian: Киста яичника (Kista yaitchnika)

- Mandarin: 卵巢囊肿 (luǎncháo nángzhòng)

- Definition: A fluid-filled sac that forms on or inside the ovary, often causing abdominal pain, bloating, or changes in menstrual cycle.

121. Gallstones

- French: Calculs biliaires

- Spanish: Cálculos biliares

- German: Gallensteine

- Russian: Желчные камни (Zheltchnyye kamni)

- Mandarin: 胆结石 (dǎn jiéshí)

- Definition: Hard deposits formed in the gallbladder or bile ducts, typically composed of cholesterol or bilirubin, causing severe abdominal pain, nausea, and vomiting.

122. Glomerulonephritis

- French: Glomérulonéphrite

- Spanish: Glomerulonefritis

- German: Glomerulonephritis

- Russian: Гломерулонефрит (Glomerulonefrit)

- Mandarin: 肾小球肾炎 (shèn xiǎoqiú shènyán)

- Definition: Inflammation of the glomeruli in the kidneys, leading to proteinuria, hematuria, and impaired kidney function.

123. Diverticulitis

- French: Diverticulite

- Spanish: Diverticulitis

- German: Divertikulitis

- Russian: Дивертикулит (Divertikulit)

- Mandarin: 憩室炎 (qìshì yán)

- Definition: Inflammation or infection of the diverticula, small pouches that can form in the lining of the digestive system, causing abdominal pain, fever, and changes in bowel habits.

124. Cirrhosis

- French: Cirrhose

- Spanish: Cirrosis

- German: Zirrhose

- Russian: Цирроз (Tsirroz)

- Mandarin: 肝硬化 (gān yìnghuà)

- Definition: Chronic liver disease characterized by the progressive scarring of liver tissue, leading to impaired liver function, jaundice, and complications such as ascites and hepatic encephalopathy.

125. Anemia

- French: Anémie

- Spanish: Anemia

- German: Anämie

- Russian: Анемия (Anemiya)

- Mandarin: 贫血 (pínxiě)

- Definition: A condition characterized by a deficiency of red blood cells or hemoglobin in the blood, leading to fatigue, weakness, and shortness of breath.

126. Appendicitis

- French: Appendicite

- Spanish: Apendicitis

- German: Appendizitis

- Russian: Аппендицит (Appenditsit)

- Mandarin: 阑尾炎 (lánwěi yán)

- Definition: Inflammation of the appendix, a small pouch attached to the large intestine, typically causing abdominal pain, nausea, vomiting, and fever.

127. Varicose veins

- French: Varices

- Spanish: Varices

- German: Krampfadern

- Russian: Варикозное расширение вен (Varikoznoye

rasshireniye ven)

- Mandarin: 静脉曲张 (jìngmài qūzhāng)

- Definition: Enlarged and twisted veins, usually appearing in the legs, that can cause pain, swelling, and aching discomfort.

128. Gastroesophageal reflux disease (GERD)

- French: Reflux gastro-œsophagien (RGO)

- Spanish: Enfermedad por reflujo gastroesofágico (ERGE)

- German: Gastroösophagealer Reflux (GERD)

- Russian: Гастроэзофагеальный рефлюкс (GERD) (Gastroezofageal'nyy reflyuks)

- Mandarin: 胃食管反流病 (wèi shíguǎn fǎnliú bìng)

- Definition: A chronic digestive disorder where stomach acid flows back into the esophagus, causing heartburn, chest pain, and discomfort.

129. Benign prostatic hyperplasia (BPH)

- French: Hyperplasie bénigne de la prostate (HBP)

- Spanish: Hiperplasia benigna de próstata (HBP)

- German: Benigne Prostatahyperplasie (BPH)

- Russian: Доброкачественная гиперплазия простаты (Dobrokachestvennaya giperplaziya prostaty)

- Mandarin: 良性前列腺增生 (liángxìng qiánlièxiàn zēngshēng)

- Definition: Non-cancerous enlargement of the prostate gland, which can cause urinary symptoms such as frequent urination, urgency, and weak urine flow.

130. Systemic lupus erythematosus (SLE)

- French: Lupus érythémateux disséminé (LED)

- Spanish: Lupus eritematoso sistémico (LES)

- German: Systemischer Lupus erythematodes (SLE)

- Russian: Системная красная волчанка (Sistemnaya krasnaya volchanka)

- Mandarin: 系统性红斑狼疮 (xìtǒngxìng hóngbān lángchuáng)

- Definition: Autoimmune disease where the immune system attacks healthy tissues, leading to inflammation and damage to various organs and systems, including joints, skin, kidneys, and heart.

131. Hypertensive heart disease

- French: Cardiopathie hypertensive

- Spanish: Cardiopatía hipertensiva

- German: Hypertensive Herzerkrankung

- Russian: Гипертоническая болезнь сердца (Gipertonicheskaya bolezn' serdtsa)

- Mandarin: 高血压性心脏病 (gāo xuèyā xìng xīnzàng bìng)

- Definition: Heart conditions caused by long-term high blood pressure, which can lead to coronary artery disease, heart failure, and other complications.

132. Interstitial cystitis

- French: Cystite interstitielle

- Spanish: Cistitis intersticial

- German: Interstitielle Zystitis

- Russian: Интерстициальный цистит (Interstitsial'nyy tsistit)

- Mandarin: 间质性膀胱炎 (jiànzhìxìng pángguāng yán)

- Definition: Chronic bladder condition characterized by pelvic pain, urinary urgency, and frequency, often without bacterial infection.

133. Chronic kidney disease (CKD)

- French: Maladie rénale chronique (MRC)

- Spanish: Enfermedad renal crónica (ERC)

- German: Chronische Nierenkrankheit (CKD)

- Russian: Хроническая болезнь почек (Khronicheskaya bolezn' pochek)

- Mandarin: 慢性肾脏病 (màn xìng shènzàng bìng)

- Definition: Progressive loss of kidney function over time, leading to complications such as fluid retention, electrolyte imbalances, and anemia.

134. Chronic obstructive pulmonary disease (COPD)

- French: Maladie pulmonaire obstructive chronique (MPOC)

- Spanish: Enfermedad pulmonar obstructiva crónica (EPOC)

- German: Chronisch obstruktive Lungenerkrankung (COPD)

- Russian: Хроническое обструктивное заболевание легких (ХОЗЛ) (Khronicheskoye obstruktivnoye zabolevaniye legkikh)

- Mandarin: 慢性阻塞性肺疾病 (màn xìng zǔ sè xìng fèi jí bìng)

- Definition: Progressive lung disease characterized by airflow limitation, usually caused by exposure to irritants such as cigarette smoke, leading to symptoms like coughing, wheezing, and shortness of breath.

135. Diabetic neuropathy

- French: Neuropathie diabétique

- Spanish: Neuropatía diabética

- German: Diabetische Neuropathie

- Russian: Диабетическая нейропатия (Diabeticheskaya neyropatiya)

- Mandarin: 糖尿病性神经病变 (tángniàobìngxìng shénjīng bìngbiàn)

- Definition: Nerve damage caused by diabetes, leading to symptoms such as numbness, tingling, and pain in the affected areas, often in the hands and feet.

9. BODY PLACES

1. Head

   - French: Tête

   - Spanish: Cabeza

   - German: Kopf

   - Russian: Голова (Golova)

   - Mandarin: 头部 (tóu bù)

   - Definition: The uppermost part of the human body, containing the brain, eyes, nose, mouth, and ears.

2. Neck

   - French: Cou

   - Spanish: Cuello

   - German: Hals

   - Russian: Шея (Shcheya)

   - Mandarin: 颈部 (jǐng bù)

   - Definition: The part of the body that connects the head to the torso, containing the cervical spine and supporting structures.

3. Shoulder

    - French: Épaule

    - Spanish: Hombro

    - German: Schulter

    - Russian: Плечо (Plecho)

    - Mandarin: 肩膀 (jiānbǎng)

    - Definition: The joint connecting the arm to the torso, allowing for a wide range of motion.

4. Arm

    - French: Bras

    - Spanish: Brazo

    - German: Arm

    - Russian: Рука (Ruka)

    - Mandarin: 手臂 (shǒu bì)

    - Definition: The upper limb of the body, extending from the shoulder to the hand.

5. Elbow

    - French: Coude

    - Spanish: Codo

    - German: Ellenbogen

    - Russian: Локоть (Lokot')

    - Mandarin: 肘部 (zhǒu bù)

    - Definition: The joint between the upper arm and the forearm, allowing for bending and straightening of the arm.

6. Forearm

   - French: Avant-bras

   - Spanish: Antebrazo

   - German: Unterarm

   - Russian: Предплечье (Predplech'ye)

   - Mandarin: 前臂 (qián bì)

   - Definition: The part of the arm between the elbow and the wrist.

7. Wrist

   - French: Poignet

   - Spanish: Muñeca

   - German: Handgelenk

   - Russian: Запястье (Zapyast'ye)

   - Mandarin: 手腕 (shǒu wàn)

   - Definition: The joint connecting the hand to the forearm, allowing for flexibility and movement.

8. Hand

   - French: Main

   - Spanish: Mano

   - German: Hand

   - Russian: Рука (Ruka)

   - Mandarin: 手 (shǒu)

   - Definition: The terminal part of the upper limb, consisting of the palm, fingers, and thumb.

9. Fingers

- French: Doigts

- Spanish: Dedos

- German: Finger

- Russian: Пальцы (Pal'tsy)

- Mandarin: 手指 (shǒu zhǐ)

- Definition: The digits of the hand, used for grasping, touching, and manipulating objects.

10. Thumb

   - French: Pouce

   - Spanish: Pulgar

   - German: Daumen

   - Russian: Большой палец (Bol'shoy palets)

   - Mandarin: 拇指 (mǔ zhǐ)

   - Definition: The first digit of the hand, opposite the fingers, allowing for grasping and fine motor movements.

11. Chest

   - French: Poitrine

   - Spanish: Pecho

   - German: Brust

   - Russian: Грудь (Grud')

   - Mandarin: 胸部 (xiōng bù)

   - Definition: The front part of the body between the neck and the abdomen, housing the heart and lungs.

12. Breast

- French: Sein

- Spanish: Seno

- German: Brust

- Russian: Грудь (Grud')

- Mandarin: 乳房 (rǔ fáng)

- Definition: Either of the two soft protruding organs on the upper front of a woman's body that secrete milk after pregnancy.

13. Back

- French: Dos

- Spanish: Espalda

- German: Rücken

- Russian: Спина (Spina)

- Mandarin: 背部 (bèi bù)

- Definition: The rear surface of the human body, extending from the neck to the pelvis.

14. Spine

- French: Colonne vertébrale

- Spanish: Columna vertebral

- German: Wirbelsäule

- Russian: Позвоночник (Pozvonochnik)

- Mandarin: 脊柱 (jízhù)

- Definition: A series of vertebrae extending from the skull to the pelvis, providing support and protection for the spinal cord.

15. Waist

- French: Taille

- Spanish: Cintura

- German: Taille

- Russian: Талия (Taliya)

- Mandarin: 腰部 (yāo bù)

- Definition: The narrowing of the body between the ribs and hips, often considered the part of the body above and including the hips.

16. Abdomen

- French: Abdomen

- Spanish: Abdomen

- German: Bauch

- Russian: Живот (Zhivot)

- Mandarin: 腹部 (fù bù)

- Definition: The area of the body containing the digestive organs, bounded by the diaphragm and pelvis.

17. Belly

- French: Ventre

- Spanish: Vientre

- German: Bauch

- Russian: Живот (Zhivot)

- Mandarin: 肚子 (dùzi)

- Definition: The front part of the abdomen, often used informally to refer to the stomach area.

18. Hip

- French: Hanche

- Spanish: Cadera

- German: Hüfte

- Russian: Бедро (Bedro)

- Mandarin: 臀部 (tún bù)

- Definition: The joint where the thigh bone meets the pelvis, providing stability and support for the body's weight.

19. Thigh

- French: Cuisse

- Spanish: Muslo

- German: Oberschenkel

- Russian: Бедро (Bedro)

- Mandarin: 大腿 (dà tuǐ)

- Definition: The part of the leg between the hip and the knee.

20. Knee

- French: Genou

- Spanish: Rodilla

- German: Knie

- Russian: Колено (Koleno)

- Mandarin: 膝盖 (xīgài)

- Definition: The joint between the thigh and the lower leg, allowing for bending and straightening movements.

31. Face

- French: Visage

- Spanish: Cara

- German: Gesicht

- Russian: Лицо (Litso)

- Mandarin: 脸 (liǎn)

- Definition: The front part of the head, including the forehead, eyes, nose, mouth, and chin.

32. Forehead

- French: Front

- Spanish: Frente

- German: Stirn

- Russian: Лоб (Lob)

- Mandarin: 前额 (qián'é)

- Definition: The part of the face above the eyebrows and between the temples.

33. Eyebrow

- French: Sourcil

- Spanish: Ceja

- German: Augenbraue

- Russian: Бровь (Brov')

- Mandarin: 眉毛 (méi máo)

- Definition: The strip of hair growing on the ridge above the eye socket.

34. Eye

- French: Œil

- Spanish: Ojo

- German: Auge

- Russian: Глаз (Glaz)

- Mandarin: 眼睛 (yǎnjing)

- Definition: The organ of sight, responsible for detecting light and transmitting signals to the brain.

35. Eyelash

- French: Cil

- Spanish: Pestaña

- German: Wimper

- Russian: Ресница (Resnitsa)

- Mandarin: 睫毛 (jiémáo)

- Definition: One of the short hairs growing on the edges of the eyelids.

36. Ear

- French: Oreille

- Spanish: Oreja

- German: Ohr

- Russian: Ухо (Ukho)

- Mandarin: 耳朵 (ěrduo)

- Definition: The organ of hearing and balance, located on each side of the head.

37. Nose

- French: Nez

- Spanish: Nariz

- German: Nase

- Russian: Нос (Nos)

- Mandarin: 鼻子 (bízi)

- Definition: The organ of smell and the primary passageway for air entering the respiratory system.

38. Nostril

- French: Narine

- Spanish: Fosa nasal

- German: Nasenloch

- Russian: Ноздря (Nozdr'ya)

- Mandarin: 鼻孔 (bíkǒng)

- Definition: One of the two external openings of the nasal cavity, allowing air to enter and exit the nose.

39. Mouth

- French: Bouche

- Spanish: Boca

- German: Mund

- Russian: Рот (Rot)

- Mandarin: 嘴 (zuǐ)

- Definition: The cavity in the face used for eating, drinking, speaking, and breathing.

40. Lips

- French: Lèvres

- Spanish: Labios

- German: Lippen

- Russian: Губы (Guby)

- Mandarin: 嘴唇 (zuǐchún)

- Definition: The two fleshy parts forming the opening of the mouth, used for speaking, eating, and expressing emotions.

41. Cheek

- French: Joue

- Spanish: Mejilla

- German: Wange

- Russian: Щека (Shcheka)

- Mandarin: 脸颊 (liǎnjiá)

- Definition: The fleshy area of the face below the eye and between the nose and ear.

42. Chin

- French: Menton

- Spanish: Barbilla

- German: Kinn

- Russian: Подбородок (Podborodok)

- Mandarin: 下巴 (xiàba)

- Definition: The prominent part of the lower face, below the lower lip.

43. Jaw

- French: Mâchoire

  - Spanish: Mandíbula

  - German: Kiefer

  - Russian: Челюсть (Chelyust')

  - Mandarin: 下颌 (xiàhé)

  - Definition: The framework of bones forming the mouth and holding the teeth, including the mandible and maxilla.

44. Teeth

  - French: Dents

  - Spanish: Dientes

  - German: Zähne

  - Russian: Зубы (Zuby)

  - Mandarin: 牙齿 (yáchǐ)

  - Definition: Hard, white structures in the mouth used for biting and chewing food.

45. Gums

  - French: Gencives

  - Spanish: Encías

  - German: Zahnfleisch

  - Russian: Десна (Desna)

  - Mandarin: 牙龈 (yáyín)

  - Definition: Soft tissue surrounding the teeth, providing support and protection for the roots.

46. Tongue

- French: Langue

   - Spanish: Lengua

   - German: Zunge

   - Russian: Язык (Yazyk)

   - Mandarin: 舌头 (shétou)

   - Definition: A muscular organ in the mouth used for tasting, swallowing, and speaking.

47. Palate

   - French: Palais

   - Spanish: Paladar

   - German: Gaumen

   - Russian: Небо (Nebo)

   - Mandarin: 上颚 (shàng'é)

   - Definition: The roof of the mouth, consisting of the hard palate and soft palate.

48. Throat

   - French: Gorge

   - Spanish: Garganta

   - German: Hals

   - Russian: Горло (Gorlo)

   - Mandarin: 喉咙 (hóulóng)

   - Definition: The passage from the mouth to the esophagus and trachea, used for swallowing and breathing.

49. Adam's apple

- French: Pomme d'Adam

- Spanish: Manzana de Adán

- German: Adamsapfel

- Russian: Яблоко Адама (Yabloko Adama)

- Mandarin: 喉结 (hóu jié)

- Definition: A prominent bulge in the throat formed by the thyroid cartilage of the larynx.

50. Larynx

   - French: Larynx

   - Spanish: Laringe

   - German: Kehlkopf

   - Russian: Гортань (Gortan')

   - Mandarin: 喉 (hóu)

   - Definition: The organ of voice production, located in the throat, containing the vocal cords.

51. Voice

   - French: Voix

   - Spanish: Voz

   - German: Stimme

   - Russian: Голос (Golos)

   - Mandarin: 声音 (shēngyīn)

   - Definition: Sound produced by vibration of the vocal cords in the larynx, used for speech and communication.

52. Tonsil

- French: Amygdale

- Spanish: Amígdala

- German: Mandel

- Russian: Миндалина (Minalina)

- Mandarin: 扁桃体 (biǎntáotǐ)

- Definition: Small masses of lymphoid tissue located at the back of the throat, involved in immune response.

53. Esophagus

- French: Œsophage

- Spanish: Esófago

- German: Speiseröhre

- Russian: Пищевод (Pishchevod)

- Mandarin: 食管 (shíguǎn)

- Definition: The muscular tube connecting the throat to the stomach, through which food passes during swallowing.

54. Stomach

- French: Estomac

- Spanish: Estómago

- German: Magen

- Russian: Желудок (Zhelyudok)

- Mandarin: 胃 (wèi)

- Definition: The organ in the abdomen where digestion of food occurs, secreting digestive enzymes and acids.

55. Liver

- French: Foie

- Spanish: Hígado

- German: Leber

- Russian: Печень (Pechen')

- Mandarin: 肝 (gān)

- Definition: A large organ in the abdomen responsible for detoxification, metabolism, and storage of nutrients.

56. Gallbladder

- French: Vésicule biliaire

- Spanish: Vesícula biliar

- German: Gallenblase

- Russian: Желчный пузырь (Zheltchnyy puzyr')

- Mandarin: 胆囊 (dǎnnáng)

- Definition: A small pouch beneath the liver that stores and concentrates bile produced by the liver.

57. Pancreas

- French: Pancréas

- Spanish: Páncreas

- German: Bauchspeicheldrüse

- Russian: Поджелудочная железа (Podzheludochnaya zheleza)

- Mandarin: 胰腺 (yí xiàn)

- Definition: An organ located behind the stomach that produces digestive enzymes and insulin.

58. Spleen

   - French: Rate

   - Spanish: Bazo

   - German: Milz

   - Russian: Селезенка (Selezenka)

   - Mandarin: 脾脏 (pí zàng)

   - Definition: An organ located in the abdomen involved in filtering blood and immune response.

59. Intestine

   - French: Intestin

   - Spanish: Intestino

   - German: Darm

   - Russian: Кишечник (Kishechnik)

   - Mandarin: 肠 (cháng)

   - Definition: The long, tube-like organ in the abdomen where digestion and absorption of nutrients occur.

60. Colon

   - French: Côlon

   - Spanish: Colon

   - German: Dickdarm

   - Russian: Толстая кишка (Tolstaya kishka)

   - Mandarin: 结肠 (jié cháng)

   - Definition: The large intestine, responsible for absorbing water and electrolytes from undigested food and forming feces.

61. Rectum

- French: Rectum

- Spanish: Recto

- German: Rektum

- Russian: Прямая кишка (Pryamaya kishka)

- Mandarin: 直肠 (zhí cháng)

- Definition: The final section of the large intestine, connecting the colon to the anus and storing feces before elimination.

62. Anus

- French: Anus

- Spanish: Ano

- German: Anus

- Russian: Анус (Anus)

- Mandarin: 肛门 (gāngmén)

- Definition: The opening at the end of the digestive tract through which feces are expelled from the body.

63. Bladder

- French: Vessie

- Spanish: Vejiga

- German: Blase

- Russian: Мочевой пузырь (Mochevoy puzyr')

- Mandarin: 膀胱 (bǎngguāng)

- Definition: A hollow muscular organ in the pelvis that stores urine before it is expelled from the body.

64. Kidney

   - French: Rein

   - Spanish: Riñón

   - German: Niere

   - Russian: Почка (Pochka)

   - Mandarin: 肾 (shèn)

   - Definition: A pair of organs located in the back of the abdomen responsible for filtering waste products from the blood to form urine.

65. Ureter

   - French: Uretère

   - Spanish: Uréter

   - German: Harnleiter

   - Russian: Мочеточник (Mochetochnik)

   - Mandarin: 输尿管 (shū niào guǎn)

   - Definition: A muscular tube that carries urine from the kidney to the bladder.

66. Urethra

   - French: Urètre

   - Spanish: Uretra

   - German: Harnröhre

   - Russian: Мочеиспускательный канал (Mocheispuskatel'nyy kanal)

   - Mandarin: 尿道 (niào dào)

- Definition: The tube that carries urine from the bladder to the outside of the body during urination.

67. Prostate

- French: Prostate

- Spanish: Próstata

- German: Prostata

- Russian: Предстательная железа (Predstatel'naya zheleza)

- Mandarin: 前列腺 (qiánlièxiàn)

- Definition: A gland in males located below the bladder, surrounding the urethra, and producing fluid that makes up part of semen.

68. Testicle

- French: Testicule

- Spanish: Testículo

- German: Hoden

- Russian: Яичко (Yaychko)

- Mandarin: 睾丸 (gāowán)

- Definition: One of the two male reproductive organs responsible for producing sperm and testosterone.

69. Ovary

- French: Ovaire

- Spanish: Ovario

- German: Eierstock

- Russian: Яичник (Yaychnik)

- Mandarin: 卵巢 (luǎncháo)

- Definition: One of the paired female reproductive organs responsible for producing eggs and hormones.

70. Uterus

  - French: Utérus

  - Spanish: Útero

  - German: Gebärmutter

  - Russian: Матка (Matka)

  - Mandarin: 子宫 (zǐgōng)

  - Definition: A hollow, muscular organ in females where fertilized eggs implant and develop into a fetus during pregnancy.

71. Vagina

  - French: Vagin

  - Spanish: Vagina

  - German: Vagina

  - Russian: Влагалище (Vlagalishche)

  - Mandarin: 阴道 (yīndào)

  - Definition: The muscular tube in females that extends from the vulva to the cervix, serving as the birth canal and allowing for menstrual flow.

72. Vulva

  - French: Vulve

  - Spanish: Vulva

  - German: Vulva

  - Russian: Вульва (Vul'va)

- Mandarin: 外阴 (wàiyīn)

- Definition: The external female genitalia, including the labia majora, labia minora, clitoris, and vaginal opening.

73. Penis

    - French: Pénis

    - Spanish: Pene

    - German: Penis

    - Russian: Пенис (Penis)

    - Mandarin: 阴茎 (yīnjīng)

    - Definition: The male organ of copulation and urination, consisting of the shaft, glans, and urethral opening.

74. Scrotum

    - French: Scrotum

    - Spanish: Escroto

    - German: Hodensack

    - Russian: Мошонка (Moshonka)

    - Mandarin: 阴囊 (yīnnáng)

    - Definition: The pouch of skin and muscle containing the testicles in males.

75. Clitoris

    - French: Clitoris

    - Spanish: Clítoris

    - German: Klitoris

    - Russian: Клитор (Klitor)

- Mandarin: 阴蒂 (yīndì)

- Definition: A small, sensitive organ located above the urethral opening in females, involved in sexual arousal and pleasure.

76. Labia

- French: Lèvres

- Spanish: Labios

- German: Schamlippen

- Russian: Половые губы (Polovyye guby)

- Mandarin: 阴唇 (yīnchún)

- Definition: The outer and inner folds of skin surrounding the vaginal opening in females.

77. Breasts

- French: Seins

- Spanish: Senos

- German: Brüste

- Russian: Грудь (Grud')

- Mandarin: 乳房 (rǔfáng)

- Definition: The mammary glands on the chest of females and males, containing milk-producing tissue.

78. Nipple

- French: Téton

- Spanish: Pezón

- German: Brustwarze

- Russian: Сосок (Sosok)

- Mandarin: 乳头 (rǔtóu)

- Definition: The raised, pigmented area of skin on the breast from which milk ducts emerge.

79. Areola

- French: Aréole

- Spanish: Areola

- German: Warzenvorhof

- Russian: Грудинка (Grudinka)

- Mandarin: 乳晕 (rǔ yūn)

- Definition: The circular area of darker skin surrounding the nipple on the breast.

80. Prostate gland

- French: Glande prostatique

- Spanish: Glándula prostática

- German: Prostata

- Russian: Предстательная железа (Predstatel'naya zheleza)

- Mandarin: 前列腺 (qiánlièxiàn)

- Definition: A gland in males located below the bladder, surrounding the urethra, and producing fluid that makes up part of semen.

81. Cervix

- French: Col de l'utérus

- Spanish: Cuello del útero

- German: Gebärmutterhals

- Russian: Шейка матки (Sheyka matki)

- Mandarin: 子宫颈 (zǐgōng jǐng)

- Definition: The lower narrow end of the uterus that connects to the vagina, serving as the passageway for menstrual blood and sperm.

82. Fallopian tube

- French: Trompe de Fallope

- Spanish: Trompa de Falopio

- German: Eileiter

- Russian: Фаллопиева труба (Fallopieva truba)

- Mandarin: 输卵管 (shū luǎn guǎn)

- Definition: One of a pair of tubes connecting the ovaries to the uterus, through which the egg travels from the ovary to the uterus.

83. Ovum

- French: Ovule

- Spanish: Óvulo

- German: Eizelle

- Russian: Яйцеклетка (Yaytseklechka)

- Mandarin: 卵子 (luǎnzǐ)

- Definition: A female reproductive cell, or egg, released by the ovary during ovulation, capable of being fertilized by sperm.

84. Umbilical cord

- French: Cordon ombilical

- Spanish: Cordón umbilical

- German: Nabelschnur

- Russian: Пуповина (Pupovina)

- Mandarin: 脐带 (qídài)

- Definition: A flexible cord containing blood vessels that connects a fetus to the placenta during gestation, providing nutrients and oxygen.

85. Placenta

- French: Placenta

- Spanish: Placenta

- German: Plazenta

- Russian: Плацента (Platzenta)

- Mandarin: 胎盘 (tāipán)

- Definition: An organ formed during pregnancy that provides oxygen and nutrients to the fetus and removes waste products from the fetus's blood.

86. Amniotic fluid

- French: Liquide amniotique

- Spanish: Líquido amniótico

- German: Fruchtwasser

- Russian: Амниотическая жидкость (Amnioticheskaya zhidkost')

- Mandarin: 羊水 (yáng shuǐ)

- Definition: The fluid surrounding the fetus within the amniotic sac, protecting the fetus from injury and helping regulate temperature.

87. Fetus

- French: Fœtus

- Spanish: Feto

- German: Fetus

- Russian: Плод (Plod)

- Mandarin: 胎儿 (tāi'ér)

- Definition: The developing human organism from the end of the eighth week after conception until birth.

88. Uterine lining

- French: Endomètre

- Spanish: Endometrio

- German: Gebärmutterschleimhaut

- Russian: Слизистая оболочка матки (Slizistaya obolochka matki)

- Mandarin: 子宫内膜 (zǐgōng nèimó)

- Definition: The inner lining of the uterus that thickens and sheds during the menstrual cycle and pregnancy.

89. Menstruation

- French: Menstruation

- Spanish: Menstruación

- German: Menstruation

- Russian: Менструация (Mestruatsiya)

- Mandarin: 月经 (yuèjīng)

- Definition: The monthly shedding of the uterine lining, typically accompanied by bleeding, in females who are not pregnant.

90. Ovulation

- French: Ovulation

- Spanish: Ovulación

- German: Ovulation

- Russian: Овуляция (Ovulyatsiya)

- Mandarin: 排卵 (páiluǎn)

- Definition: The release of a mature egg from the ovary, typically occurring midway through the menstrual cycle.

91. Ejaculation

- French: Éjaculation

- Spanish: Eyaculación

- German: Ejakulation

- Russian: Эякуляция (Eyakulyatsiya)

- Mandarin: 射精 (shèjīng)

- Definition: The release of semen from the male reproductive tract, typically during orgasm.

92. Fertilization

- French: Fécondation

- Spanish: Fertilización

- German: Befruchtung

- Russian: Оплодотворение (Oplodotvoreniye)

- Mandarin: 受精 (shòujīng)

- Definition: The union of a sperm cell and an egg cell, resulting in the formation of a zygote.

93. Conception

- French: Conception

   - Spanish: Concepción

   - German: Empfängnis

   - Russian: Зачатие (Zachatye)

   - Mandarin: 受孕 (shòuyùn)

   - Definition: The moment when fertilization occurs, leading to the beginning of pregnancy.

94. Gestation

   - French: Gestation

   - Spanish: Gestación

   - German: Schwangerschaft

   - Russian: Беременность (Beremennost')

   - Mandarin: 妊娠 (rènshēn)

   - Definition: The period of time during which a fetus develops inside the uterus, typically lasting around nine months in humans.

95. Labor

   - French: Accouchement

   - Spanish: Parto

   - German: Geburt

   - Russian: Роды (Rody)

   - Mandarin: 分娩 (fēnmiǎn)

   - Definition: The process of childbirth, including contractions of the uterus, dilation of the cervix, and expulsion of the fetus and placenta.

96. Delivery

- French: Accouchement

- Spanish: Parto

- German: Geburt

- Russian: Роды (Rody)

- Mandarin: 分娩 (fēnmiǎn)

- Definition: The act of giving birth to a baby.

97. Postpartum

- French: Postpartum

- Spanish: Postparto

- German: Postpartal

- Russian: Послеродовой (Poslerodovoy)

- Mandarin: 产后 (chǎnhòu)

- Definition: Relating to the period of time following childbirth, typically up to six weeks after delivery.

98. Prenatal

- French: Prénatal

- Spanish: Prenatal

- German: Pränatal

- Russian: Пренатальный (Prenatal'nyy)

- Mandarin: 产前 (chǎnqián)

- Definition: Relating to the period before birth, especially referring to medical care and development during pregnancy.

99. Neonatal

- French: Néonatal

- Spanish: Neonatal

- German: Neonatal

- Russian: Новорожденный (Novorozhdennyy)

- Mandarin: 新生儿 (xīnshēng'ér)

- Definition: Relating to newborn infants, typically referring to the first month after birth.

100. Infant

- French: Bébé

- Spanish: Bebé

- German: Säugling

- Russian: Младенец (Mladenets)

- Mandarin: 婴儿 (yīng'ér)

- Definition: A very young child, especially one who is not yet able to walk or talk.

101. Pediatrics

- French: Pédiatrie

- Spanish: Pediatría

- German: Pädiatrie

- Russian: Педиатрия (Pediatriya)

- Mandarin: 小儿科 (xiǎo ér kē)

- Definition: The branch of medicine that deals with the medical care of infants, children, and adolescents.

102. Childhood

- French: Enfance

- Spanish: Infancia

- German: Kindheit

- Russian: Детство (Detstvo)

- Mandarin: 童年 (tóngnián)

- Definition: The period of life between infancy and adolescence, typically lasting from birth to puberty.

103. Adolescence

- French: Adolescence

- Spanish: Adolescencia

- German: Adoleszenz

- Russian: Подростковый возраст (Podrostkovyy vozrast)

- Mandarin: 青春期 (qīngchūn qī)

- Definition: The transitional stage of physical and psychological development between childhood and adulthood, typically beginning with puberty.

104. Growth

- French: Croissance

- Spanish: Crecimiento

- German: Wachstum

- Russian: Рост (Rost)

- Mandarin: 生长 (shēngzhǎng)

- Definition: The process of increasing in physical size and development, typically measured in height and weight.

105. Development

- French: Développement

- Spanish: Desarrollo

- German: Entwicklung

- Russian: Развитие (Razvitiye)

- Mandarin: 发育 (fāyù)

- Definition: The process of growth, maturation, and learning that occurs throughout life, involving physical, cognitive, and emotional changes.

106. Milestone

- French: Jalon

- Spanish: Hitos

- German: Meilenstein

- Russian: Веха (Vekha)

- Mandarin: 里程碑 (lǐchéngbēi)

- Definition: An important event or achievement that marks a significant point in development or progress.

107. Motor skills

- French: Motricité

- Spanish: Habilidades motoras

- German: Motorische Fähigkeiten

- Russian: Моторные навыки (Motornyye navyki)

- Mandarin: 运动技能 (yùndòng jìnéng)

- Definition: The ability to control and coordinate movements of the body, including both gross motor skills (large movements) and fine motor skills (small movements).

108. Cognitive development

- French: Développement cognitif

- Spanish: Desarrollo cognitivo

- German: Kognitive Entwicklung

- Russian: Когнитивное развитие (Kognitivnoye razvitiye)

- Mandarin: 认知发展 (rènzhī fāzhǎn)

- Definition: The process of acquiring knowledge, understanding, and problem-solving abilities, typically involving memory, language, and reasoning skills.

109. Language acquisition

- French: Acquisition du langage

- Spanish: Adquisición del lenguaje

- German: Spracherwerb

- Russian: Приобретение языка (Priobreteniye yazyka)

- Mandarin: 语言习得 (yǔyán xídé)

- Definition: The process by which humans acquire the capacity to perceive and comprehend language, as well as to produce and use words and sentences to communicate.

110. Socialization

- French: Socialisation

- Spanish: Socialización

- German: Sozialisation

- Russian: Социализация (Sotsializatsiya)

- Mandarin: 社会化 (shèhuì huà)

- Definition: The process of learning and internalizing the values, norms, and behaviors of a society, typically through interactions with others and cultural experiences.

10. SO HOT! FEVERS

1. Fever

   - French: Fièvre

   - Spanish: Fiebre

   - German: Fieber

   - Russian: Жар (Zhar)

   - Mandarin: 发烧 (Fāshāo)

   - Definition: Abnormal elevation of body temperature, often indicating an underlying illness or infection.

2. Cough

   - French: Toux

   - Spanish: Tos

   - German: Husten

   - Russian: Кашель (Kashel')

   - Mandarin: 咳嗽 (Késòu)

   - Definition: Forceful expulsion of air from the lungs typically due to irritation or infection of the airways.

3. Headache

   - French: Mal de tête

   - Spanish: Dolor de cabeza

- German: Kopfschmerzen

- Russian: Головная боль (Golovnaya bol')

- Mandarin: 头痛 (Tóutòng)

- Definition: Pain in the head or upper neck region, can vary in intensity and duration.

4. Nausea

- French: Nausée

- Spanish: Náuseas

- German: Übelkeit

- Russian: Тошнота (Toshnota)

- Mandarin: 恶心 (Ěxīn)

- Definition: Feeling of discomfort in the stomach with an inclination to vomit, often a precursor to vomiting.

5. Vomiting

- French: Vomissement

- Spanish: Vómito

- German: Erbrechen

- Russian: Рвота (Rvota)

- Mandarin: 呕吐 (Ōutù)

- Definition: Forceful expulsion of stomach contents through the mouth, often due to illness or irritation.

6. Diarrhea

- French: Diarrhée

- Spanish: Diarrea

- German: Durchfall

- Russian: Понос (Ponos)

- Mandarin: 腹泻 (Fùxiè)

- Definition: Frequent passage of loose or watery stools, often indicating gastrointestinal distress.

7. Rash

- French: Éruption cutanée

- Spanish: Erupción cutánea

- German: Hautausschlag

- Russian: Сыпь (Syp')

- Mandarin: 皮疹 (Pízhěn)

- Definition: Change in the skin's appearance, often characterized by redness, itching, and inflammation.

8. Fatigue

- French: Fatigue

- Spanish: Fatiga

- German: Müdigkeit

- Russian: Усталость (Ustalost')

- Mandarin: 疲劳 (Píláo)

- Definition: Feeling of extreme tiredness or exhaustion, often persistent and interfering with daily activities.

9. Dizziness

- French: Étourdissement

- Spanish: Mareo

- German: Schwindel

- Russian: Головокружение (Golovokruzheniye)

- Mandarin: 头晕 (Tóuyūn)

- Definition: Sensation of lightheadedness or unsteadiness, often accompanied by a spinning feeling.

10. Shortness of breath

   - French: Essoufflement

   - Spanish: Falta de aliento

   - German: Atemnot

   - Russian: Одышка (Odyshka)

   - Mandarin: 呼吸困难 (Hūxī kùnnán)

   - Definition: Difficulty in breathing, often characterized by a sensation of not getting enough air.

11. Chest pain

   - French: Douleur thoracique

   - Spanish: Dolor en el pecho

   - German: Brustschmerz

   - Russian: Боль в груди (Bol' v grudi)

   - Mandarin: 胸痛 (Xiōngtòng)

   - Definition: Pain or discomfort felt in the chest region, which may vary in intensity and duration.

12. Sore throat

   - French: Mal de gorge

   - Spanish: Dolor de garganta

- German: Halsschmerzen

   - Russian: Боль в горле (Bol' v gorle)

   - Mandarin: 喉咙痛 (Hóulóng tòng)

   - Definition: Pain, scratchiness, or irritation of the throat, often worsened by swallowing.

13. Stomachache

   - French: Mal de ventre

   - Spanish: Dolor de estómago

   - German: Bauchschmerzen

   - Russian: Боль в животе (Bol' v zhivote)

   - Mandarin: 胃痛 (Wèitòng)

   - Definition: Pain or discomfort felt in the abdominal region, often associated with digestive issues.

14. Swelling

   - French: Gonflement

   - Spanish: Hinchazón

   - German: Schwellung

   - Russian: Отёк (Otyok)

   - Mandarin: 肿胀 (Zhǒngzhàng)

   - Definition: Enlargement or puffiness of a body part typically due to fluid accumulation.

15. Bruise

   - French: Contusion

   - Spanish: Moretón

- German: Bluterguss

- Russian: Синяк (Sinyak)

- Mandarin: 淤青 (Yūqīng)

- Definition: Discoloration of the skin caused by bleeding underneath due to an impact or injury.

16. Itching

   - French: Démangeaison

   - Spanish: Picazón

   - German: Juckreiz

   - Russian: Зуд (Zud)

   - Mandarin: 痒 (Yǎng)

- Definition: Uncomfortable sensation on the skin that causes an urge to scratch.

17. Joint pain

   - French: Douleur articulaire

   - Spanish: Dolor articular

   - German: Gelenkschmerzen

   - Russian: Боль в суставе (Bol' v sustave)

   - Mandarin: 关节痛 (Guānjié tòng)

- Definition: Pain or discomfort felt in the joints, often associated with inflammation or injury.

18. Constipation

   - French: Constipation

   - Spanish: Estreñimiento

- German: Verstopfung

- Russian: Запор (Zapor)

- Mandarin: 便秘 (Biànmì)

- Definition: Difficulty in passing stools or infrequent bowel movements.

19. Blood pressure

- French: Pression artérielle

- Spanish: Presión arterial

- German: Blutdruck

- Russian: Артери

20. Palpitations

- French: Palpitations

- Spanish: Palpitaciones

- German: Herzrasen

- Russian: Пальпитации (Pal'pitatsii)

- Mandarin: 心悸 (Xīnjì)

- Definition: Awareness of one's heartbeat, often characterized by rapid, irregular, or pounding sensations in the chest.

21. Urinary urgency

- French: Urgence urinaire

- Spanish: Urgencia urinaria

- German: Harnwegsprobleme

- Russian: Срочное мочеиспускание (Srochnoye mocheispuskaniye)

  - Mandarin: 尿急 (Niào jí)

  - Definition: Strong, sudden need to urinate immediately.

22. Urinary frequency

    - French: Fréquence urinaire

    - Spanish: Frecuencia urinaria

    - German: Harnfrequenz

    - Russian: Частое мочеиспускание (Chastoye mocheispuskaniye)

    - Mandarin: 排尿频率 (Páiniào pínlǜ)

    - Definition: Increased need to urinate more often than usual.

23. Polyuria

    - French: Polyurie

    - Spanish: Poliuria

    - German: Polyurie

    - Russian: Полиурия (Poliuriya)

    - Mandarin: 多尿 (Duō niào)

    - Definition: Excessive production of urine, leading to increased frequency and volume of urination.

24. Polydipsia

    - French: Polydipsie

    - Spanish: Polidipsia

    - German: Polydipsie

    - Russian: Полидипсия (Polidipsiya)

- Mandarin: 多饮 (Duō yǐn)

- Definition: Excessive thirst, often associated with dehydration or certain medical conditions.

25. Dysphagia

- French: Dysphagie

- Spanish: Disfagia

- German: Dysphagie

- Russian: Дисфагия (Disfagiya)

- Mandarin: 吞咽困难 (Tūnyàn kùnnán)

- Definition: Difficulty or discomfort in swallowing food or liquids.

26. Hematuria

- French: Hématurie

- Spanish: Hematuria

- German: Hämaturie

- Russian: Гематурия (Gematuriya)

- Mandarin: 血尿 (Xiě niào)

- Definition: Presence of blood in the urine, which may indicate various underlying conditions.

27. Hemoptysis

- French: Hémoptysie

- Spanish: Hemoptisis

- German: Hämoptoe

- Russian: Гемоптоз (Gemoptoz)

- Mandarin: 咯血 (Géli)

- Definition: Coughing up blood from the respiratory tract, often associated with lung or bronchial disorders.

28. Hematemesis

- French: Hématémèse

- Spanish: Hematemesis

- German: Hämatemesis

- Russian: Гематемез (Gematemiez)

- Mandarin: 吐血 (Tùxiě)

- Definition: Vomiting blood, usually originating from the upper gastrointestinal tract.

29. Melena

- French: Mélenas

- Spanish: Melena

- German: Meläna

- Russian: Мелена (Melena)

- Mandarin: 黑便 (Hēibiàn)

- Definition: Black, tarry stool resulting from the presence of digested blood, typically from upper gastrointestinal bleeding.

30. Anorexia

- French: Anorexie

- Spanish: Anorexia

- German: Anorexie

- Russian: Анорексия (Anoreksiya)

- Mandarin: 厌食 (Yànshí)

- Definition: Loss of appetite or disinterest in food consumption, often associated with underlying medical or psychological factors.

31. Constipation

- French: Constipation

- Spanish: Estreñimiento

- German: Verstopfung

- Russian: Запор (Zapor)

- Mandarin: 便秘 (Biànmì)

- Definition: Difficulty in passing stools or infrequent bowel movements.

32. Incontinence

- French: Incontinence

- Spanish: Incontinencia

- German: Inkontinenz

- Russian: Недержание (Nederzhaniye)

- Mandarin: 失禁 (Shījìn)

- Definition: Inability to control bladder or bowel movements, leading to involuntary leakage.

33. Hemorrhage

- French: Hémorragie

- Spanish: Hemorragia

- German: Blutung

- Russian: Кровотечение (Krovotecheniye)

- Mandarin: 出血 (Chūxiě)

- Definition: Profuse bleeding, either internally or externally, from ruptured blood vessels.

34. Seizure

　- French: Crise

　- Spanish: Convulsión

　- German: Anfall

　- Russian: Припадок (Pripadok)

　- Mandarin: 发作 (Fāzuò)

- Definition: Sudden, uncontrolled electrical disturbance in the brain, resulting in abnormal behavior, movements, or sensations.

35. Syncope

　- French: Syncope

　- Spanish: Síncope

　- German: Ohnmacht

　- Russian: Синкопа (Sinkopa)

　- Mandarin: 晕厥 (Yūnjué)

- Definition: Temporary loss of consciousness due to a lack of blood flow to the brain; also known as fainting.

36. Insomnia

　- French: Insomnie

　- Spanish: Insomnio

　- German: Schlaflosigkeit

　- Russian: Бессонница (Bessonnitsa)

- Mandarin: 失眠 (Shīmián)

- Definition: Difficulty falling asleep or staying asleep, leading to inadequate rest and daytime fatigue.

37. Apnea

   - French: Apnée

   - Spanish: Apnea

   - German: Apnoe

   - Russian: Апноэ (Apnoe)

   - Mandarin: 呼吸暂停 (Hūxī zàntíng)

   - Definition: Temporary cessation of breathing, often occurring during sleep.

38. Tinnitus

   - French: Acouphène

   - Spanish: Tinnitus

   - German: Tinnitus

   - Russian: Звон в ушах (Zvon v ushakh)

   - Mandarin: 耳鸣 (Ěrmíng)

   - Definition: Perception of noise or ringing in the ears, not caused by external sound sources.

39. Vertigo

   - French: Vertige

   - Spanish: Vértigo

   - German: Schwindel

   - Russian: Головокружение (Golovokruzheniye)

- Mandarin: 眩晕 (Xuànyūn)

- Definition: Sensation of spinning or dizziness, often with a feeling of imbalance.

40. Pallor

   - French: Pâleur

   - Spanish: Palidez

   - German: Blässe

   - Russian: Бледность (Blednost')

   - Mandarin: 苍白 (Cāngbái)

- Definition: Unnatural paleness or lack of color in the skin, often indicating illness, shock, or emotional distress.

41. Edema

   - French: Œdème

   - Spanish: Edema

   - German: Ödem

   - Russian: Отёк (Otyok)

   - Mandarin: 水肿 (Shuǐzhǒng)

- Definition: Swelling caused by fluid retention in tissues, often due to an underlying medical condition.

42. Hypertension

   - French: Hypertension

   - Spanish: Hipertensión

- German: Hypertonie

- Russian: Гипертония (Gipertoniya)

- Mandarin: 高血压 (Gāo xuèyā)

- Definition: High blood pressure, a condition where the force of blood against artery walls is consistently too high.

43. Hypotension

- French: Hypotension

- Spanish: Hipotensión

- German: Hypotonie

- Russian: Гипотония (Gipotoniya)

- Mandarin: 低血压 (Dī xuèyā)

- Definition: Low blood pressure, a condition where the force of blood against artery walls is consistently too low.

44. Hyperglycemia

- French: Hyperglycémie

- Spanish: Hiperglucemia

- German: Hyperglykämie

- Russian: Гипергликемия (Giperglikemiya)

- Mandarin: 高血糖 (Gāo xuètáng)

- Definition: Elevated levels of glucose (sugar) in the blood, often associated with diabetes or other metabolic disorders.

45. Hypoglycemia

- French: Hypoglycémie

- Spanish: Hipoglucemia

- German: Hypoglykämie

- Russian: Гипогликемия (Gipoglikemiya)

- Mandarin: 低血糖 (Dī xuètáng)

- Definition: Abnormally low levels of glucose (sugar) in the blood, which can lead to symptoms such as weakness, sweating, and confusion.

46. Hyperthermia

- French: Hyperthermie

- Spanish: Hipertermia

- German: Hyperthermie

- Russian: Гипертермия (Gipertermiya)

- Mandarin: 体温过高 (Tǐwēn guògāo)

- Definition: Elevated body temperature beyond the normal range, often caused by external heat exposure or medical conditions.

47. Hypothermia

- French: Hypothermie

- Spanish: Hipotermia

- German: Hypothermie

- Russian: Гипотермия (Gipotermiya)

- Mandarin: 体温过低 (Tǐwēn guòdī)

- Definition: Abnormally low body temperature, typically caused by exposure to cold temperatures.

48. Arrhythmia

- French: Arythmie

- Spanish: Arritmia

- German: Arrhythmie

- Russian: Аритмия (Aritmiya)

- Mandarin: 心律不齐 (Xīnlǜ bùqí)

- Definition: Abnormal heart rhythm, characterized by irregular or erratic beating of the heart.

49. Palpitation

- French: Palpitation

- Spanish: Palpitación

- German: Herzrasen

- Russian: Пальпитация (Pal'pitatsiya)

- Mandarin: 心悸 (Xīnjì)

- Definition: Awareness of one's heartbeat, often characterized by rapid, irregular, or pounding sensations in the chest.

50. Cyanosis

- French: Cyanose

- Spanish: Cianosis

- German: Zyanose

- Russian: Цианоз (Tsiyanoz)

- Mandarin: 发绀 (Fāgàn)

- Definition: Bluish discoloration of the skin or mucous membranes due to inadequate oxygenation of the blood.

51. Anemia

- French: Anémie

- Spanish: Anemia

- German: Anämie

- Russian: Анемия (Anemiya)

- Mandarin: 贫血 (Pínxiě)

- Definition: Condition characterized by a deficiency of red blood cells or hemoglobin, leading to reduced oxygen transport to tissues and organs.

52. Leukocytosis

- French: Leucocytose

- Spanish: Leucocitosis

- German: Leukozytose

- Russian: Лейкоцитоз (Leykotsitoz)

- Mandarin: 白细胞增多 (Báixìbāo zēngduō)

- Definition: Elevated white blood cell count, often indicating an immune response to infection or inflammation.

53. Leukopenia

- French: Leucopénie

- Spanish: Leucopenia

- German: Leukopenie

- Russian: Лейкопения (Leykopeniya)

- Mandarin: 白细胞减少 (Báixìbāo jiǎnshǎo)

- Definition: Abnormally low white blood cell count, which can increase the risk of infections.

54. Thrombocytopenia

- French: Thrombopénie

- Spanish: Trombocitopenia

- German: Thrombozytopenie

- Russian: Тромбоцитопения (Trombotsitopeniya)

- Mandarin: 血小板减少 (Xuè xiǎobǎn jiǎnshǎo)

- Definition: Decrease in the number of platelets in the blood, leading to impaired blood clotting and an increased risk of bleeding.

55. Hemoglobin

- French: Hémoglobine

- Spanish: Hemoglobina

- German: Hämoglobin

- Russian: Гемоглобин (Gemoglobin)

- Mandarin: 血红蛋白 (Xiěhóng dànbái)

- Definition: Protein in red blood cells that carries oxygen from the lungs to the body's tissues and organs.

56. Serum

- French: Sérum

- Spanish: Suero

- German: Serum

- Russian: Сыворотка (Syvorotka)

- Mandarin: 血清 (Xiěqīng)

- Definition: Clear, yellowish fluid portion of blood that remains after blood has clotted, containing various proteins, electrolytes, hormones, and antibodies.

57. Electrocardiogram (ECG or EKG)

- French: Électrocardiogramme (ECG ou EKG)

- Spanish: Electrocardiograma (ECG o EKG)

- German: Elektrokardiogramm (EKG)

- Russian: Электрокардиограмма (Elektrokardiogramma)

- Mandarin: 心电图 (Xīndiàntú)

- Definition: Graphic representation of the electrical activity of the heart over a period of time, used to diagnose various heart conditions.

58. Ultrasound

- French: Échographie

- Spanish: Ecografía

- German: Ultraschall

- Russian: Ультразвук (Ultrazvuk)

- Mandarin: 超声波 (Chāoshēng bō)

- Definition: Imaging technique that uses high-frequency sound waves to produce images of structures within the body, commonly used for diagnostic purposes.

59. Magnetic Resonance Imaging (MRI)

- French: Imagerie par résonance magnétique (IRM)

- Spanish: Imagen por resonancia magnética (IRM)

- German: Magnetresonanztomographie (MRT)

- Russian: Магнитно-резонансная томография (Magnitno-rezonansnaya tomografiya)

- Mandarin: 磁共振成像 (Cí gòngzhèn chéngxiàng)

Definition: Imaging technique that uses strong magnetic fields and radio waves to generate detailed images of the internal structures of the body.

60. Computed Tomography (CT or CAT scan)

- French: Tomodensitométrie (TDM ou scanner)

- Spanish: Tomografía computarizada (TC o escáner)

- German: Computertomographie (CT oder CAT-Scan)

- Russian: Компьютерная томография (Komp'yuternaya tomografiya)

- Mandarin: 计算机断层扫描 (Jìsuànjī duàncéng sǎomiáo)

- Definition: Imaging technique that uses X-rays and computer processing to create detailed cross-sectional images of the body's internal structures.

61. Biopsy

- French: Biopsie

- Spanish: Biopsia

- German: Biopsie

- Russian: Биопсия (Biopsiya)

- Mandarin: 活检 (Huó jiǎn)

- Definition: Surgical procedure to remove a small sample of tissue for examination under a microscope, often used to diagnose diseases such as cancer.

62. Endoscopy

- French: Endoscopie

- Spanish: Endoscopia

- German: Endoskopie

- Russian: Эндоскопия (Endoskopiya)

- Mandarin: 内窥镜检查 (Nèi kuī jìng jiǎnchá)

  - Definition: Medical procedure that uses a flexible tube with a light and camera to visualize the interior of organs or cavities within the body, often used for diagnostic or therapeutic purposes.

63. Colonoscopy

  - French: Colonoscopie

  - Spanish: Colonoscopia

  - German: Koloskopie

  - Russian: Колоноскопия (Kolonoskopiya)

  - Mandarin: 结肠镜检查 (Jiécháng jìng jiǎnchá)

  - Definition: Endoscopic examination of the large intestine (colon) and the rectum, often used to screen for colorectal cancer or diagnose gastrointestinal conditions.

64. Bronchoscopy

  - French: Bronchoscopie

  - Spanish: Broncoscopia

  - German: Bronchoskopie

  - Russian: Бронхоскопия (Bronkhoskopiya)

  - Mandarin: 支气管镜检查 (Zhī qìguǎn jìng jiǎnchá)

  - Definition: Endoscopic examination of the bronchial tubes (airways) within the lungs, often used to diagnose respiratory conditions or retrieve tissue samples.

65. Laparoscopy

  - French: Laparoscopie

  - Spanish: Laparoscopia

- German: Laparoskopie

- Russian: Лапароскопия (Laparoskopiya)

- Mandarin: 腹腔镜检查 (Fùqiāng jìng jiǎnchá)

- Definition: Surgical procedure that uses a thin, lighted tube (laparoscope) inserted through a small incision in the abdomen to visualize and perform operations within the abdominal cavity.

66. Lumbar puncture (Spinal tap)

- French: Ponction lombaire (Ponction rachidienne)

- Spanish: Punción lumbar (Punción espinal)

- German: Lumbalpunktion (Spinalpunktion)

- Russian: Пункция спинного мозга (Punktsiya spinnogo mozga)

- Mandarin: 腰椎穿刺 (Yāozhuī chuānchī)

- Definition: Medical procedure that involves inserting a needle into the spinal canal to collect cerebrospinal fluid for diagnostic or therapeutic purposes.

67. Electroencephalogram (EEG)

- French: Électroencéphalogramme (EEG)

- Spanish: Electroencefalograma (EEG)

- German: Elektroenzephalogramm (EEG)

- Russian: Электроэнцефалограмма (Elektroentsefalogramma)

- Mandarin: 脑电图 (Nǎodiàntú)

- Definition: Recording of the electrical activity of the brain, typically using electrodes placed on the scalp, used to diagnose various neurological conditions.

68. Spirometry

- French: Spirométrie

- Spanish: Espirometría

- German: Spirometrie

- Russian: Спирометрия (Spirometriya)

- Mandarin: 肺功能检查 (Fèi gōngnéng jiǎnchá)

- Definition: Test that measures the volume of air inspired and expired by the lungs, used to assess lung function and diagnose respiratory conditions such as asthma or chronic obstructive pulmonary disease (COPD).

69. Arthroscopy

- French: Arthroscopie

- Spanish: Artroscopia

- German: Arthroskopie

- Russian: Артроскопия (Artroskopiya)

- Mandarin: 关节镜检查 (Guānjié jìng jiǎnchá)

- Definition: Minimally invasive surgical procedure that uses a small camera (arthroscope) inserted into a joint through a small incision to visualize and treat joint problems.

70. Mammography

- French: Mammographie

- Spanish: Mamografía

- German: Mammographie

- Russian: Маммография (Mammografiya)

- Mandarin: 乳房X线摄影 (Rǔfáng X xiàn shèyǐng)

- Definition: Imaging technique that uses low-dose X-rays to visualize and detect abnormalities in the breast tissue, often used for breast cancer screening.

71. Histopathology

   - French: Histopathologie

   - Spanish: Histopatología

   - German: Histopathologie

   - Russian: Гистопатология (Gistopatologiya)

   - Mandarin: 组织病理学 (Zǔzhī bìnglǐxué)

   - Definition: Study of diseased tissues at a microscopic level to diagnose diseases and understand their cellular and tissue changes.

72. Radiography

   - French: Radiographie

   - Spanish: Radiografía

   - German: Radiographie

   - Russian: Рентгенография (Rentgenografiya)

   - Mandarin: X线摄影 (X xiàn shèyǐng)

   - Definition: Imaging technique that uses X-rays to produce images of the internal structures of the body, commonly used for diagnostic purposes.

73. Nuclear Medicine

   - French: Médecine nucléaire

   - Spanish: Medicina nuclear

   - German: Nuklearmedizin

- Russian: Ядерная медицина (Yadernaya meditsina)

- Mandarin: 核医学 (Hé yīxué)

- Definition: Medical specialty that uses radioactive substances to diagnose and treat diseases, such as cancer and thyroid disorders.

74. Angiography

- French: Angiographie

- Spanish: Angiografía

- German: Angiographie

- Russian: Ангиография (Angiografiya)

- Mandarin: 血管造影术 (Xiěguǎn zàoyǐng shù)

- Definition: Imaging technique that uses X-rays and a contrast dye to visualize the blood vessels and their flow within the body, often used to diagnose vascular conditions.

75. Fluoroscopy

- French: Fluoroscopie

- Spanish: Fluoroscopia

- German: Fluoroskopie

- Russian: Флюороскопия (Flyuoroskopiya)

- Mandarin: 透视 (Tòushì)

- Definition: Real-time imaging technique that uses X-rays to capture moving images of the internal structures of the body, commonly used during medical procedures such as surgeries and catheter placements.

76. Tomosynthesis

- French: Tomosynthèse

- Spanish: Tomosíntesis

- German: Tomosynthese

- Russian: Томосинтез (Tomosintez)

- Mandarin: 层析摄影术 (Céng xī shèyǐng shù)

- Definition: Imaging technique that creates three-dimensional images of the breast tissue using multiple X-ray images taken at different angles, often used for breast cancer screening.

77. Positron Emission Tomography (PET scan)

   - French: Tomographie par émission de positons (TEP)

   - Spanish: Tomografía por emisión de positrones (PET)

   - German: Positronen-Emissions-Tomographie (PET)

   - Russian: Позитронно-эмиссионная томография (Pozitronno-emissionnaya tomografiya)

   - Mandarin: 正电子发射断层扫描 (Zhèngdiànzi fāshè duàncéng sǎomiáo)

   - Definition: Imaging technique that uses a radioactive tracer to detect metabolic activity and function in tissues and organs, commonly used for cancer diagnosis and staging.

78. Bone Density Scan (DEXA scan)

   - French: Scintigraphie osseuse (DEXA)

   - Spanish: Densitometría ósea (DEXA)

   - German: Knochendichtemessung (DEXA)

   - Russian: Денситометрия костей (DEXA)

   - Mandarin: 骨密度扫描 (Gǔ mìdù sǎomiáo)

   - Definition: Imaging technique that measures bone mineral density to assess bone health and diagnose conditions such as osteoporosis.

79. Thermography

- French: Thermographie

- Spanish: Termografía

- German: Thermographie

- Russian: Термография (Termografiya)

- Mandarin: 热像术 (Rè xiàng shù)

- Definition: Imaging technique that uses infrared radiation to detect and visualize temperature variations in the body, often used for detecting inflammation, vascular disorders, and breast abnormalities.

80. Magnetic Resonance Angiography (MRA)

- French: Angiographie par résonance magnétique (ARM)

- Spanish: Angiografía por resonancia magnética (ARM)

- German: Magnetresonanzangiographie (MRA)

- Russian: Магнитно-резонансная ангиография (Magnetno-rezonansnaya angiografiya)

- Mandarin: 磁共振血管造影 (Cí gòngzhèn xuèguǎn zàoyǐng)

- Definition: Imaging technique that uses magnetic resonance imaging (MRI) to visualize blood vessels and blood flow within the body, often used to diagnose vascular conditions such as aneurysms and stenosis.

81. Magnetic Resonance Cholangiopancreatography (MRCP)

- French: Cholangiopancréatographie par résonance magnétique (MRCP)

- Spanish: Colangiopancreatografía por resonancia magnética (MRCP)

- German: Magnetresonanz-Cholangiopankreatikographie (MRCP)

- Russian: Магнитно-резонансная холангиопанкреатография (MRCP)

- Mandarin: 磁共振胆胰管造影 (Cí gòngzhèn dǎn yí guǎn zàoyǐng)

- Definition: Imaging technique that uses magnetic resonance imaging (MRI) to visualize the bile ducts and pancreatic ducts, often used to diagnose conditions such as gallstones, tumors, and pancreatitis.

82. Sigmoidoscopy

- French: Sigmoidoscopie

- Spanish: Sigmoidoscopia

- German: Sigmoidoskopie

- Russian: Сигмоидоскопия (Sigmoidoskopiya)

- Mandarin: 结肠镜检查 (Jiécháng jìng jiǎnchá)

- Definition: Endoscopic examination of the sigmoid colon, the lower part of the large intestine, often used to screen for colorectal cancer or diagnose gastrointestinal conditions.

83. Ophthalmoscopy

- French: Ophtalmoscopie

- Spanish: Oftalmoscopia

- German: Ophthalmoskopie

- Russian: Офтальмоскопия (Oftalmoskopiya)

- Mandarin: 眼底检查 (Yǎndǐ jiǎnchá)

- Definition: Examination of the interior structures of the eye, such as the retina, optic nerve, and blood vessels, using a device called an ophthalmoscope.

84. Otoscopy

　- French: Otoscopie

　- Spanish: Otoscopia

　- German: Otoskopie

　- Russian: Отоскопия (Otoskopiya)

　- Mandarin: 耳镜检查 (Ěr jìng jiǎnchá)

- Definition: Examination of the ear canal and eardrum using a device called an otoscope, often used to diagnose ear infections, earwax buildup, or other ear conditions.

85. Cystoscopy

　- French: Cystoscopie

　- Spanish: Cistoscopia

　- German: Zystoskopie

　- Russian: Цистоскопия (Tsistoskopiya)

　- Mandarin: 膀胱镜检查 (Pángguāng jìng jiǎnchá)

- Definition: Endoscopic examination of the bladder and urethra, often used to diagnose urinary tract conditions such as bladder cancer, urinary stones, or urinary incontinence.

86. Laryngoscopy

　- French: Laryngoscopie

　- Spanish: Laringoscopia

　- German: Laryngoskopie

　- Russian: Ларингоскопия (Laringoskopiya)

- Mandarin: 喉镜检查 (Hóu jìng jiǎnchá)

- Definition: Endoscopic examination of the larynx (voice box) and vocal cords, often used to diagnose voice disorders, throat conditions, or perform biopsies.

87. Hysteroscopy

- French: Hystéroscopie

- Spanish: Histeroscopia

- German: Hysteroskopie

- Russian: Гистероскопия (Gisteroskopiya)

- Mandarin: 子宫镜检查 (Zǐgōng jìng jiǎnchá)

- Definition: Endoscopic examination of the uterus and cervix, often used to diagnose and treat conditions such as abnormal bleeding, fibroids, or polyps.

88. Esophagogastroduodenoscopy (EGD)

- French: Endoscopie digestive haute (EGD)

- Spanish: Endoscopia digestiva alta (EGD)

- German: Ösophagogastroduodenoskopie (EGD)

- Russian: Эзофагогастродуоденоскопия (EZOGDS)

- Mandarin: 食管胃十二指肠镜检查 (Shíguǎn wèi shí'èr zhǐcháng jìng jiǎnchá)

- Definition: Endoscopic examination of the esophagus, stomach, and duodenum (first part of the small intestine), often used to diagnose gastrointestinal conditions such as ulcers, gastritis, or reflux disease.

89. Gastroscopy

- French: Gastroscopie

- Spanish: Gastroscopia

- German: Gastroskopie

- Russian: Гастроскопия (Gastroskopiya)

- Mandarin: 胃镜检查 (Wèi jìng jiǎnchá)

- Definition: Endoscopic examination of the stomach, often used to diagnose conditions such as ulcers, inflammation, or tumors.

90. Colposcopy

- French: Colposcopie

- Spanish: Colposcopia

- German: Kolposkopie

- Russian: Кольпоскопия (Kol'poskopiya)

- Mandarin: 阴道镜检查 (Yīndào jìng jiǎnchá)

- Definition: Visual examination of the cervix and vagina using a device called a colposcope, often used to detect abnormal cells or lesions that may indicate cervical cancer or other gynecological conditions.

91. Audiometry

- French: Audiométrie

- Spanish: Audiometría

- German: Audiometrie

- Russian: Аудиометрия (Audiometriya)

- Mandarin: 听力测试 (Tīnglì cèshì)

- Definition: Test that measures hearing sensitivity and ability to perceive sounds of different frequencies, often used to diagnose hearing loss or assess hearing function.

92. Electroencephalography (EEG)

- French: Électroencéphalographie (EEG)

- Spanish: Electroencefalografía (EEG)

- German: Elektroenzephalographie (EEG)

- Russian: Электроэнцефалография (Elektroentsefalografiya)

- Mandarin: 脑电图检查 (Nǎodiàntú jiǎnchá)

- Definition: Recording of the electrical activity of the brain, typically using electrodes placed on the scalp, used to diagnose various neurological conditions.

93. Electromyography (EMG)

- French: Électromyographie (EMG)

- Spanish: Electromiografía (EMG)

- German: Elektromyographie (EMG)

- Russian: Электромиография (Elektromiografiya)

- Mandarin: 肌电图检查 (Jīdiàntú jiǎnchá)

- Definition: Recording of the electrical activity of muscles, typically using electrodes inserted into the muscle tissue, used to diagnose neuromuscular disorders or assess muscle function.

94. Polysomnography (PSG)

- French: Polysomnographie (PSG)

- Spanish: Polisomnografía (PSG)

- German: Polysomnographie (PSG)

- Russian: Полисомнография (Polisomnografiya)

- Mandarin: 多导睡眠图检查 (Duō dǎo shuìmián tú jiǎnchá)

- Definition: Recording of multiple physiological parameters during sleep, such as brain waves, heart rate, breathing, and muscle activity, used to diagnose sleep disorders such as sleep apnea or insomnia.

95. Pulmonary Function Test (PFT)

- French: Test de la fonction pulmonaire (PFT)

- Spanish: Prueba de función pulmonar (PFT)

- German: Lungenfunktionstest (PFT)

- Russian: Функциональные тесты легких (PFT)

- Mandarin: 肺功能测试 (Fèi gōngnéng cèshì)

- Definition: Series of tests that measure lung function, including lung capacity, airflow, and gas exchange, used to diagnose respiratory conditions such as asthma, chronic obstructive pulmonary disease (COPD), or restrictive lung diseases.

96. Cardiac Stress Test

- French: Test de stress cardiaque

- Spanish: Prueba de esfuerzo cardíaco

- German: Herzbelastungstest

- Russian: Кардиологическое нагрузочное тестирование

- Mandarin: 心脏应激测试 (Xīnzàng yìngjī cèshì)

- Definition: Test that measures the heart's ability to respond to stress or exercise, often using electrocardiography (ECG) or imaging techniques, used to diagnose coronary artery disease or evaluate heart function.

97. Holter Monitor

- French: Moniteur Holter

- Spanish: Monitor Holter

- German: Holter-Monitor

- Russian: Монитор Холтера

- Mandarin: Holter 监测器 (Holter jiāncè qì)

- Definition: Portable device that continuously records the heart's electrical activity over a period of 24 to 48 hours, used to diagnose cardiac arrhythmias or assess heart function.

98. Ambulatory Blood Pressure Monitoring (ABPM)

- French: Monitorage ambulatoire de la pression artérielle (MAPA)

- Spanish: Monitorización ambulatoria de la presión arterial (MAPA)

- German: Ambulantes Blutdruckmonitoring (ABDM)

- Russian: Амбулаторное мониторирование артериального давления (АМАД)

- Mandarin: 动态血压监测 (Dòngtài xuèyā jiāncè)

- Definition: Method of measuring blood pressure at regular intervals over a 24-hour period, often using a portable device worn by the patient, used to diagnose hypertension or assess blood pressure variations throughout the day.

99. Pulse Oximetry

- French: Oxymétrie de pouls

- Spanish: Oximetría de pulso

- German: Pulsoxymetrie

- Russian: Пульсоксиметрия

- Mandarin: 脉搏血氧饱和度检测 (Màibó xuèyǎng bǎohédù jiǎncè)

- Definition: Non-invasive method of monitoring oxygen saturation in the blood by measuring the percentage of hemoglobin saturated with oxygen, often using a small device attached to a finger or earlobe.

100. Body Mass Index (BMI)

- French: Indice de masse corporelle (IMC)

- Spanish: Índice de masa corporal (IMC)

- German: Body-Mass-Index (BMI)

- Russian: Индекс массы тела (ИМТ)

- Mandarin: 身体质量指数 (Shēntǐ zhìliàng zhǐshù)

- Definition: Measure of body fat based on height and weight, calculated by dividing weight in kilograms by the square of height in meters, used to assess whether an individual is underweight, normal weight, overweight, or obese.

101. Body Temperature

- French: Température corporelle

- Spanish: Temperatura corporal

- German: Körpertemperatur

- Russian: Температура тела

- Mandarin: 体温 (Tǐwēn)

- Definition: Measure of the body's internal heat level, typically measured using a thermometer, with the normal range around 36.5–37.5 degrees Celsius (97.7–99.5 degrees Fahrenheit).

102. Blood Pressure

- French: Pression artérielle

- Spanish: Presión arterial

- German: Blutdruck

- Russian: Артериальное давление

- Mandarin: 血压 (Xiěyā)

- Definition: Force exerted by circulating blood against the walls of blood vessels, typically measured using a sphygmomanometer, with a normal range around 120/80 mmHg.

103. Heart Rate

- French: Fréquence cardiaque

- Spanish: Frecuencia cardíaca

- German: Herzfrequenz

- Russian: Пульс

- Mandarin: 心率 (Xīnlǜ)

- Definition: Number of heartbeats per minute, typically measured by counting the pulse, with the normal range around 60–100 beats per minute at rest.

104. Respiratory Rate

- French: Fréquence respiratoire

- Spanish: Frecuencia respiratoria

- German: Atemfrequenz

- Russian: Частота дыхания

- Mandarin: 呼吸频率 (Hūxī pínlǜ)

- Definition: Number of breaths taken per minute, typically measured by observing chest movements, with the normal range around 12–20 breaths per minute at rest.

105. Oxygen Saturation

   - French: Saturation en oxygène

   - Spanish: Saturación de oxígeno

   - German: Sauerstoffsättigung

   - Russian: Насыщение кислородом

   - Mandarin: 血氧饱和度 (Xiěyǎng bǎohédù)

   - Definition: Percentage of hemoglobin saturated with oxygen in the blood, typically measured using pulse oximetry, with the normal range around 95–100%.

106. Glucose Level

   - French: Niveau de glucose

   - Spanish: Nivel de glucosa

   - German: Glukosespiegel

   - Russian: Уровень глюкозы

   - Mandarin: 葡萄糖水平 (Pútáotáng shuǐpíng)

   - Definition: Concentration of glucose (sugar) in the blood, typically measured using a blood glucose meter, with the normal fasting range around 70–100 mg/dL (3.9–5.6 mmol/L).

107. Cholesterol Level

   - French: Niveau de cholestérol

   - Spanish: Nivel de colesterol

   - German: Cholesterinspiegel

   - Russian: Уровень холестерина

   - Mandarin: 胆固醇水平 (Dǎn gùchún shuǐpíng)

   - Definition: Concentration of cholesterol in the blood, typically measured as total cholesterol, LDL (low-density lipoprotein), HDL (high-density lipoprotein), and triglycerides.

108. White Blood Cell Count

- French: Numération des globules blancs

- Spanish: Recuento de glóbulos blancos

- German: Anzahl der weißen Blutkörperchen

- Russian: Уровень лейкоцитов

- Mandarin: 白细胞计数 (Báixìbāo jìshǔ)

- Definition: Number of white blood cells per volume of blood, typically measured using a blood test, with the normal range around 4,000–11,000 cells per microliter.

109. Red Blood Cell Count

- French: Numération des globules rouges

- Spanish: Recuento de glóbulos rojos

- German: Anzahl der roten Blutkörperchen

- Russian: Уровень эритроцитов

- Mandarin: 红细胞计数 (Hóng xìbāo jìshǔ)

- Definition: Number of red blood cells per volume of blood, typically measured using a blood test, with the normal range around 4.2–5.4 million cells per microliter for men and 3.6–5.0 million cells per microliter for women.

110. Platelet Count

- French: Numération plaquettaire

- Spanish: Recuento de plaquetas

- German: Thrombozytenzahl

- Russian: Уровень тромбоцитов

- Mandarin: 血小板计数 (Xiě xiǎobǎn jìshǔ)

- Definition: Number of platelets (thrombocytes) per volume of blood, typically measured using a blood test, with the normal range around 150,000 to 400,000 platelets per microliter.

111. Urine Analysis

- French: Analyse d'urine

- Spanish: Análisis de orina

- German: Urinanalyse

- Russian: Анализ мочи

- Mandarin: 尿液分析 (Niàoyè fēnxī)

- Definition: Laboratory examination of urine to assess various aspects of health, including kidney function, hydration status, presence of infections, and metabolic disorders.

112. Electrocardiogram (ECG or EKG)

- French: Électrocardiogramme (ECG ou EKG)

- Spanish: Electrocardiograma (ECG o EKG)

- German: Elektrokardiogramm (EKG)

- Russian: Электрокардиограмма (ЭКГ)

- Mandarin: 心电图检查 (Xīndiàntú jiǎnchá)

- Definition: Recording of the electrical activity of the heart, typically measured using electrodes placed on the skin, used to diagnose cardiac arrhythmias, ischemia, or structural abnormalities.

113. Blood Urea Nitrogen (BUN)

- French: Azote uréique sanguin (AUS)

- Spanish: Nitrógeno ureico en sangre (NUS)

- German: Harnstoff im Blut (HIB)

- Russian: Азот крови мочевины (АКМ)

- Mandarin: 血尿素氮 (Xiě niàosù dàn)

- Definition: Measure of the amount of urea nitrogen in the blood, used to assess kidney function and hydration status, with the normal range around 7–20 mg/dL.

114. Creatinine Level

- French: Niveau de créatinine

- Spanish: Nivel de creatinina

- German: Kreatininwert

- Russian: Уровень креатинина

- Mandarin: 肌酐水平 (Jīgǎn shuǐpíng)

- Definition: Concentration of creatinine in the blood, used as an indicator of kidney function, with the normal range around 0.6–1.3 mg/dL for men and 0.5–1.1 mg/dL for women.

115. Blood Gas Analysis

- French: Analyse de gaz sanguins

- Spanish: Análisis de gases en sangre

- German: Blutgasanalyse

- Russian: Анализ крови на газы

- Mandarin: 血气分析 (Xiěqì fēnxī)

- Definition: Laboratory test that measures the levels of oxygen, carbon dioxide, and pH in arterial blood, used to assess respiratory and metabolic status.

116. Prothrombin Time (PT)

- French: Temps de prothrombine (TP)

- Spanish: Tiempo de protrombina (TP)

- German: Prothrombinzeit (PTZ)

- Russian: Протромбиновое время (ПТВ)

- Mandarin: 凝血酶原时间 (Níngxiě méiyuán shíjiān)

- Definition: Measure of the time it takes for blood to clot, used to assess the integrity of the coagulation cascade and monitor anticoagulant therapy, with the normal range around 11–13 seconds.

117. International Normalized Ratio (INR)

- French: Taux international normalisé (INR)

- Spanish: Índice normalizado internacional (INR)

- German: International Normalized Ratio (INR)

- Russian: Международное нормализованное отношение (INR)

- Mandarin: 国际标准化比值 (Guójì biāozhǔnhuà bǐzhí)

- Definition: Standardized measure of the prothrombin time, used to monitor the effectiveness of anticoagulant therapy, with the normal range typically kept between 2.0 and 3.0 for most indications.

118. Troponin Level

- French: Niveau de troponine

- Spanish: Nivel de troponina

- German: Troponinwert

- Russian: Уровень тропонина

- Mandarin: 肌钙蛋白水平 (Jī gài dànbái shuǐpíng)

- Definition: Concentration of troponin, a protein found in cardiac muscle, measured in the blood to diagnose heart attacks or other cardiac-related conditions.

119. C-reactive Protein (CRP)

   - French: Protéine C réactive (CRP)

   - Spanish: Proteína C reactiva (PCR)

   - German: C-reaktives Protein (CRP)

   - Russian: С-реактивный белок (CRP)

   - Mandarin: C-反应蛋白 (C-fǎnyìng dànbái)

   - Definition: Marker of inflammation in the body, measured in the blood to assess the presence and severity of inflammatory conditions.

120. Hemoglobin A1c (HbA1c)

   - French: Hémoglobine A1c (HbA1c)

   - Spanish: Hemoglobina A1c (HbA1c)

   - German: Hämoglobin A1c (HbA1c)

   - Russian: Гемоглобин A1c (HbA1c)

   - Mandarin: 糖化血红蛋白 (Tánghuà xiěhóng dànbái)

   - Definition: Measure of average blood glucose levels over the past 2-3 months, used to assess long-term blood sugar control in individuals with diabetes.

121. Thyroid-stimulating Hormone (TSH)

   - French: Hormone thyréostimulante (TSH)

   - Spanish: Hormona estimulante de la tiroides (TSH)

   - German: Thyreotropin (TSH)

   - Russian: Тиреотропный гормон (ТТГ)

   - Mandarin: 促甲状腺激素 (Cù jiǎzhuàngxiàn jīsù)

- Definition: Hormone produced by the pituitary gland that stimulates the thyroid gland to produce thyroid hormones, measured in the blood to diagnose thyroid disorders.

122. Prostate-specific Antigen (PSA)

   - French: Antigène spécifique de la prostate (PSA)

   - Spanish: Antígeno específico de la próstata (PSA)

   - German: Prostataspezifisches Antigen (PSA)

   - Russian: Простатаспецифический антиген (ПСА)

   - Mandarin: 前列腺特异性抗原 (Qiánlièxiàn tèyìxìng kàngyuán)

   - Definition: Protein produced by the prostate gland, measured in the blood to screen for prostate cancer or monitor its progression.

123. Alpha-fetoprotein (AFP)

   - French: Alpha-fœtoprotéine (AFP)

   - Spanish: Alfa-fetoproteína (AFP)

   - German: Alpha-Fetoprotein (AFP)

   - Russian: Альфа-фетопротеин (АФП)

   - Mandarin: α-胎儿蛋白 (α Tāi'ér dànbái)

   - Definition: Protein produced by the liver and yolk sac of a developing fetus, measured in the blood to screen for certain fetal abnormalities or diagnose liver cancer.

124. Carcinoembryonic Antigen (CEA)

   - French: Antigène carcinoembryonnaire (ACE)

   - Spanish: Antígeno carcinoembrionario (CEA)

   - German: Karzinoembryonales Antigen (CEA)

   - Russian: Карциноэмбриональный антиген (СЭА)

- Mandarin: 癌胚抗原 (Ái péi kàngyuán)

- Definition: Protein produced by certain types of cancer cells, measured in the blood to monitor cancer treatment response or detect cancer recurrence.

125. Human Chorionic Gonadotropin (hCG)

- French: Gonadotrophine chorionique humaine (hCG)

- Spanish: Gonadotropina coriónica humana (hCG)

- German: Humanes Choriongonadotropin (hCG)

- Russian: Хорионический гонадотропин (hCG)

- Mandarin: 人绒毛膜促性腺激素 (Rén róngmáo mó cù xìngxiàn jīsù)

- Definition: Hormone produced during pregnancy, measured in the blood or urine to confirm pregnancy or diagnose certain conditions such as ectopic pregnancy or testicular cancer.

126. Alanine Aminotransferase (ALT)

- French: Alanine aminotransférase (ALAT)

- Spanish: Alanina aminotransferasa (ALT)

- German: Alanin-Aminotransferase (ALT)

- Russian: Аланинаминотрансфераза (АЛТ)

- Mandarin: 丙氨酸氨基转移酶 (Bǐng ānsuān ānjī zhuǎnyí méi)

- Definition: Enzyme found primarily in the liver, measured in the blood to assess liver function and diagnose liver diseases.

127. Aspartate Aminotransferase (AST)

- French: Aspartate aminotransférase (ASAT)

- Spanish: Aspartato aminotransferasa (AST)

- German: Aspartat-Aminotransferase (AST)

- Russian: Аспартатаминотрансфераза (АСТ)

- Mandarin: 天冬氨酸氨基转移酶 (Tiān dōng ānsuān ānjī zhuǎnyí méi)

- Definition: Enzyme found in various tissues including the heart and liver, measured in the blood to assess heart and liver function.

128. Gamma-glutamyl Transferase (GGT)

- French: Gamma-glutamyltransférase (GGT)

- Spanish: Gamma-glutamil transferasa (GGT)

- German: Gamma-Glutamyltransferase (GGT)

- Russian: Гамма-глутамилтрансфераза (ГГТ)

- Mandarin: γ-谷氨酰转移酶 (γ-Gǔānxiān zhuǎnyí méi)

- Definition: Enzyme found in the liver, pancreas, and other tissues, measured in the blood to assess liver and bile duct function.

129. Lipase

- French: Lipase

- Spanish: Lipasa

- German: Lipase

- Russian: Липаза

- Mandarin: 脂肪酶 (Zhīfáng méi)

- Definition: Enzyme produced by the pancreas to aid in the digestion of fats, measured in the blood to diagnose pancreatitis or other pancreatic disorders.

130. Amylase

- French: Amylase

- Spanish: Amilasa

- German: Amylase

- Russian: Амилаза

- Mandarin: 淀粉酶 (Diànfěn méi)

- Definition: Enzyme produced by the pancreas and salivary glands to aid in the digestion of carbohydrates, measured in the blood to diagnose pancreatitis or other pancreatic disorders.

131. Total Protein

- French: Protéines totales

- Spanish: Proteínas totales

- German: Gesamtprotein

- Russian: Общий белок

- Mandarin: 总蛋白 (Zǒng dànbái)

- Definition: Measure of the total amount of proteins in the blood, including albumin and globulins, used to assess nutritional status and liver or kidney function.

132. Albumin

- French: Albumine

- Spanish: Albúmina

- German: Albumin

- Russian: Альбумин

- Mandarin: 白蛋白 (Bái dànbái)

- Definition: Main protein produced by the liver, measured in the blood to assess liver function and nutritional status.

133. Bilirubin

- French: Bilirubine

- Spanish: Bilirrubina

- German: Bilirubin

- Russian: Билирубин

- Mandarin: 胆红素 (Dǎnhóngsù)

- Definition: Orange-yellow pigment produced during the breakdown of red blood cells, measured in the blood to assess liver function and diagnose conditions such as jaundice.

141. Erythrocyte Sedimentation Rate (ESR)

- French: Vitesse de sédimentation érythrocytaire (VSE)

- Spanish: Velocidad de sedimentación globular (VSG)

- German: Erythrozytensedimentationsrate (ESR)

- Russian: Скорость оседания эритроцитов (СОЭ)

- Mandarin: 红细胞沉降率 (Hóng xìbāo chénjiàng lǜ)

- Definition: Measure of the rate at which red blood cells settle in a tube of blood, used as a non-specific indicator of inflammation or infection.

142. Thyroid Hormones (T3, T4)

- French: Hormones thyroïdiennes (T3, T4)

- Spanish: Hormonas tiroideas (T3, T4)

- German: Schilddrüsenhormone (T3, T4)

- Russian: Гормоны щитовидной железы (T3, T4)

- Mandarin: 甲状腺激素 (T3, T4)

- Definition: Hormones produced by the thyroid gland that regulate metabolism and other body functions, measured in the blood to diagnose thyroid disorders.

143. Follicle-stimulating Hormone (FSH)

   - French: Hormone folliculostimulante (FSH)

   - Spanish: Hormona folículo estimulante (FSH)

   - German: Follikelstimulierendes Hormon (FSH)

   - Russian: Фолликулостимулирующий гормон (ФСГ)

   - Mandarin: 促卵泡激素 (Cù luǎnfāo jīsù)

   - Definition: Hormone produced by the pituitary gland that regulates reproductive processes, measured in the blood to assess fertility or diagnose reproductive disorders.

144. Luteinizing Hormone (LH)

   - French: Hormone lutéinisante (LH)

   - Spanish: Hormona luteinizante (LH)

   - German: Luteinisierendes Hormon (LH)

   - Russian: Лютеинизирующий гормон (ЛГ)

   - Mandarin: 黄体生成素 (Huángtǐ chéngshēng sù)

   - Definition: Hormone produced by the pituitary gland that regulates reproductive processes, measured in the blood to assess fertility or diagnose reproductive disorders.

145. Prolactin

   - French: Prolactine

   - Spanish: Prolactina

   - German: Prolaktin

   - Russian: Пролактин

- Mandarin: 催乳素 (Cuīrǔ sù)

- Definition: Hormone produced by the pituitary gland that stimulates milk production in breastfeeding women, measured in the blood to assess fertility or diagnose reproductive disorders.

146. Testosterone

   - French: Testostérone

   - Spanish: Testosterona

   - German: Testosteron

   - Russian: Тестостерон

   - Mandarin: 睾酮 (Gāotóng)

- Definition: Male sex hormone produced primarily in the testicles, measured in the blood to assess fertility or diagnose hormonal disorders in both men and women.

147. Estrogen

   - French: Œstrogène

   - Spanish: Estrógeno

   - German: Östrogen

   - Russian: Эстроген

   - Mandarin: 雌激素 (Cí jīsù)

- Definition: Female sex hormone produced primarily in the ovaries, measured in the blood to assess fertility or diagnose hormonal disorders in both women and men.

148. Progesterone

   - French: Progestérone

   - Spanish: Progesterona

- German: Progesteron

  - Russian: Прогестерон

  - Mandarin: 孕酮 (Yùntóng)

- Definition: Hormone produced primarily in the ovaries that plays a key role in the menstrual cycle and pregnancy, measured in the blood to assess fertility or diagnose hormonal disorders.

149. Parathyroid Hormone (PTH)

  - French: Hormone parathyroïdienne (PTH)

  - Spanish: Hormona paratiroidea (PTH)

  - German: Parathormon (PTH)

  - Russian: Паратгормон (ПТГ)

  - Mandarin: 甲状旁腺激素 (Jiǎ zhuàng páng xiàn jīsù)

- Definition: Hormone produced by the parathyroid glands that regulates calcium and phosphorus levels in the blood, measured to assess calcium metabolism and diagnose disorders such as hyperparathyroidism or hypoparathyroidism.

150. Cortisol

  - French: Cortisol

  - Spanish: Cortisol

  - German: Cortisol

  - Russian: Кортизол

  - Mandarin: 美卓尔 (Měi zhuó ěr)

- Definition: Steroid hormone produced by the adrenal glands in response to stress, measured in the blood or saliva to assess adrenal function and diagnose conditions such as Addison's disease or Cushing's syndrome.

151. Adrenocorticotropic Hormone (ACTH)

 - French: Hormone adrénocorticotrope (ACTH)

 - Spanish: Hormona adrenocorticotropa (ACTH)

 - German: Adrenocorticotropes Hormon (ACTH)

 - Russian: Адренокортикотропный гормон (ACTH)

 - Mandarin: 肾上腺皮质激素 (Shèn shàngxiàn pízhì jīsù)

 - Definition: Hormone produced by the pituitary gland that stimulates the adrenal glands to produce cortisol, measured in the blood to assess adrenal function and diagnose disorders such as adrenal insufficiency or Cushing's syndrome.

152. Growth Hormone (GH)

 - French: Hormone de croissance (GH)

 - Spanish: Hormona del crecimiento (GH)

 - German: Wachstumshormon (GH)

 - Russian: Гормон роста (ГГ)

 - Mandarin: 生长激素 (Shēngzhǎng jīsù)

 - Definition: Hormone produced by the pituitary gland that stimulates growth and cell reproduction, measured in the blood to assess growth disorders or monitor growth hormone therapy.

153. Insulin

 - French: Insuline

 - Spanish: Insulina

 - German: Insulin

 - Russian: Инсулин

 - Mandarin: 胰岛素 (Yí dǎo sù)

- Definition: Hormone produced by the pancreas that regulates blood sugar levels by facilitating the uptake of glucose into cells, measured in the blood to diagnose diabetes or monitor diabetes management.

154. Anti-Mullerian Hormone (AMH)

   - French: Hormone anti-Müllérienne (AMH)

   - Spanish: Hormona anti-Mülleriana (AMH)

   - German: Anti-Müller-Hormon (AMH)

   - Russian: Антимюллеров гормон (АМГ)

   - Mandarin: 抗米勒管激素 (Kàng mǐlè guǎn jīsù)

   - Definition: Hormone produced by ovarian follicles, measured in the blood to assess ovarian reserve and predict fertility potential.

155. Antidiuretic Hormone (ADH)

   - French: Hormone antidiurétique (ADH)

   - Spanish: Hormona antidiurética (ADH)

   - German: Antidiuretisches Hormon (ADH)

   - Russian: Антидиуретический гормон (АДГ)

   - Mandarin: 抗利尿激素 (Kàng lìniào jīsù)

   - Definition: Hormone produced by the hypothalamus and released by the pituitary gland that regulates water balance by reducing urine output, measured in the blood to assess water balance and diagnose disorders such as diabetes insipidus.

156. Aldosterone

   - French: Aldostérone

   - Spanish: Aldosterona

   - German: Aldosteron

- Russian: Альдостерон

- Mandarin: 醛固酮 (Quán gù tóng)

- Definition: Hormone produced by the adrenal glands that regulates sodium and potassium levels in the blood and helps maintain blood pressure, measured in the blood to assess adrenal function and diagnose disorders such as Addison's disease or Conn's syndrome.

157. Calcitonin

- French: Calcitonine

- Spanish: Calcitonina

- German: Calcitonin

- Russian: Кальцитонин

- Mandarin: 降钙素 (Jiàng gài sù)

- Definition: Hormone produced by the thyroid gland that helps regulate calcium levels in the blood, measured in the blood to assess calcium metabolism and diagnose conditions such as hypercalcemia or hypocalcemia.

158. Oxytocin

- French: Ocytocine

- Spanish: Oxitocina

- German: Oxytocin

- Russian: Окситоцин

- Mandarin: 催产素 (Cuī chǎn sù)

- Definition: Hormone produced by the hypothalamus and released by the pituitary gland that plays a role in childbirth, breastfeeding, and social bonding, measured in the blood to assess labor progress or diagnose disorders such as uterine inertia.

159. Follicle-stimulating Hormone (FSH)

   - French: Hormone folliculostimulante (FSH)

   - Spanish: Hormona folículo estimulante (FSH)

   - German: Follikelstimulierendes Hormon (FSH)

   - Russian: Фолликулостимулирующий гормон (ФСГ)

   - Mandarin: 促卵泡激素 (Cù luǎnfāo jīsù)

   - Definition: Hormone produced by the pituitary gland that regulates reproductive processes, measured in the blood to assess fertility or diagnose reproductive disorders.

160. Luteinizing Hormone (LH)

   - French: Hormone lutéinisante (LH)

   - Spanish: Hormona luteinizante (LH)

   - German: Luteinisierendes Hormon (LH)

   - Russian: Лютеинизирующий гормон (ЛГ)

   - Mandarin: 黄体生成素 (Huángtǐ chéngshēng sù)

   - Definition: Hormone produced by the pituitary gland that regulates reproductive processes, measured in the blood to assess fertility or diagnose reproductive disorders.

161. Prolactin

   - French: Prolactine

   - Spanish: Prolactina

   - German: Prolaktin

   - Russian: Пролактин

- Mandarin: 催乳素 (Cuīrǔ sù)

- Definition: Hormone produced by the pituitary gland that stimulates milk production in breastfeeding women, measured in the blood to assess fertility or diagnose reproductive disorders.

162. Testosterone

- French: Testostérone

- Spanish: Testosterona

- German: Testosteron

- Russian: Тестостерон

- Mandarin: 睾酮 (Gāotóng)

- Definition: Male sex hormone produced primarily in the testicles, measured in the blood to assess fertility or diagnose hormonal disorders in both men and women.

163. Estrogen

- French: Œstrogène

- Spanish: Estrógeno

- German: Östrogen

- Russian: Эстроген

- Mandarin: 雌激素 (Cí jīsù)

- Definition: Female sex hormone produced primarily in the ovaries, measured in the blood to assess fertility or diagnose hormonal disorders in both women and men.

164. Progesterone

- French: Progestérone

- Spanish: Progesterona

- German: Progesteron

- Russian: Прогестерон

- Mandarin: 孕酮 (Yùntóng)

- Definition: Hormone produced primarily in the ovaries that plays a key role in the menstrual cycle and pregnancy, measured in the blood to assess fertility or diagnose hormonal disorders.

165. Parathyroid Hormone (PTH)

- French: Hormone parathyroïdienne (PTH)

- Spanish: Hormona paratiroidea (PTH)

- German: Parathormon (PTH)

- Russian: Паратгормон (ПТГ)

- Mandarin: 甲状旁腺激素 (Jiǎ zhuàng páng xiàn jīsù)

- Definition: Hormone produced by the parathyroid glands that regulates calcium and phosphorus levels in the blood, measured to assess calcium metabolism and diagnose disorders such as hyperparathyroidism or hypoparathyroidism.

About the Author:

Eric Engle is really into languages and thought he was too stupid to be a doctor. He was wrong. He was however to clumsy to be a surgeon, blame ambliopia, it does distort depth perception and large hands which would be no good at suturing. He did however do well in his military first aid courses.

I really hope this book is useful to someone in need which is why i priced it as low as possible. Stay fit, eat well (let your food be your medicine), exercise, and try to be a moral person avoiding alcohol, tobacco, sugar (it's everywhere) and of course narcotics. These things wreck health.

Smoking cessation causes headaches mainly because tobacco elevates blood pressure greatly, so if you need to quit smoking be sure to drink lots of water, take lots of caffeine, and exercise rigorously to get the headaches under control while your blood pressure adjusts back to normal. An ounce of prevention is worth a pound of cure.

If you liked this book and want to see my other writings none of which have anything to do with medicine https://amazon.com/author/quizmaster if you would 5 star this book I would be really grateful. I only produced languages I know with fluency, not languages I am learning or have dabbled in, so I can verify that indeed these words are accurate. Here is the review link.

https://www.amazon.com/review/create-review/ref=cm_cr_othr_d_wr_but_top?ie=UTF8&channel=glance-detail&asin=B0D7FNJMSV

Thank you for healing others, for a fun quote to close:

Physician, heal thyself!

-Eric

www.ingramcontent.com/pod-product-compliance
Lightning Source LLC
Chambersburg PA
CBHW071917210526
45479CB00002B/447